The Smart-Carb Guide to Eating Out

Fast-Food & Family Restaurants

· · · · · ·

Tracy Jones, M.S.

AVERY
A MEMBER OF PENGUIN GROUP (USA) INC.
NEW YORK

Published by the Penguin Group
Penguin Group (USA) Inc., 375 Hudson Street, New York, New York 10014, USA ·
Penguin Group (Canada), 10 Alcorn Avenue, Toronto, Ontario, Canada M4V 3B2
(a division of Pearson Penguin Canada Inc.) · Penguin Books Ltd, 80 Strand,
London WC2R 0RL, England · Penguin Ireland, 25 St Stephen's Green, Dublin 2,
Ireland (a division of Penguin Books Ltd) · Penguin Group (Australia),
250 Camberwell Road, Camberwell, Victoria 3124, Australia (a division of Pearson
Australia Group Pty Ltd) · Penguin Books India Pvt Ltd, 11 Community Centre,
Panchsheel Park, New Delhi–110 017, India · Penguin Group (NZ), Cnr Airborne
and Rosedale Roads, Albany, Auckland 1310, New Zealand (a division of Pearson
New Zealand Ltd) · Penguin Books (South Africa) (Pty) Ltd, 24 Sturdee Avenue,
Rosebank, Johannesburg 2196, South Africa · Penguin Books Ltd, Registered
Offices: 80 Strand, London WC2R 0RL, England

Library of Congress Cataloging-in-Publication Data

Jones, Tracy, M.S.
The smart-carb guide to eating out : fast-food & family restaurants / Tracy Jones.
p.   cm.
Includes index.
ISBN 1-58333-209-X
1. Reducing diets.   2. Fast food restaurants.   3. Chain restaurants.   4.
Food—Composition—Tables.   5. Insulin resistance.—I. Title.
RM222.2.J626   2004   2004058542
613.2'5—dc22

Printed in the United States of America
10 9 8 7 6 5 4 3 2 1

Book design by Lovedog Studio

Neither the author nor the publisher is engaged in rendering professional advice
or services to the individual reader. The ideas, procedures, and suggestions in this
book are not intended as a substitute for consulting a physician. All matters regarding
health require medical supervision. Neither the author nor the publisher shall be
liable or responsible for any loss, injury, or damage allegedly arising from any
information or suggestion in this book. The opinions expressed in this book represent
the personal views of the author and not of the publisher.

While the author has made every effort to provide accurate telephone numbers
and Internet addresses at the time of publication, neither the publisher nor the author
assumes any responsibility for errors, or for changes that occur after publication.

Most Avery books are available at special quantity discounts for bulk purchase
for sales promotions, premiums, fund-raising, and educational needs. Special books
or book excerpts also can be created to fit specific needs. For details, write Penguin
Group (USA) Inc. Special Markets, 375 Hudson Street, New York, NY 10014.

This book is dedicated to my late grandmother Mollie Jones, who was a guiding light on health and nutrition to our family and everyone she met—not to mention, *a real smart cookie!* And to my late uncle Toby Jones, whose love of people and belief in his own spirit live on within and continue to inspire everyone he knew.

Acknowledgments

With much respect and gratitude, thank you to Dr. Barry Sears for improving the lives of countless people, including my own, with his ingenious Zone Diet and nutritional technologies. Equal gratitude goes to my mother, Margie Jones-Hausman, who taught me about the Zone Diet years ago and who has been a brilliant behind-the-scenes organizer and activist for *The Smart-Carb Guide*. An *enormous* thank-you to Barbara Howard, who helped tremendously with many aspects of the book's creation. Thank you to Yfat Reiss, who, with her expertise in marketing, publishing, and writing, brought this book to the world. Thanks to Kevin Poon for his loving inspiration and guidance. Thanks to Lowell Hausman (www.VegaWebsites.com), who created the user-friendly *SmartCarbLife* website. Thank you to my stepfather, Jeffrey Hausman, who contributed greatly to the entire project from the beginning. Thanks to Debbie Puente for being such an inspirational writing mentor and for providing invaluable suggestions and advice. *Big* thank-yous go to the wonderful people who contributed to *The Smart-Carb Guide* in many ways: Joan Kallet, Carol Goldman, Joseph Matheny, Kevin Nunnally, my sister Elana Jones, my father Don Jones, my brother Mike Jones, Dr. Claudia Santucci, Dr. Joe DiTomaso, Dr. Ellen Sutter, attorney Bob Ashen, Paula Liu, my loving friends in the Cooking Club, and Teresa at the South Davis McDonald's for brightening everyone's day!

Contents

Foreword by Barry Sears, Ph.D.
    author of *The Zone*   xi

Author's Note   xv

Chapter 1: Can You Lose Weight by
    Eating Fast Food?   1

Chapter 2: How to Lose Weight Eating
    Smart-Carb Meals   23

Chapter 3: Smart-Carb Women's Meals   55

Chapter 4: Smart-Carb Men's Meals   171

Appendix A: How *Smart-Carb Guide* Meals
    Are Calculated   279

Appendix B: Determining Fruit Size   283

Index   287

The 7-Day Quick-Start Diet for Women   299

The 7-Day Quick-Start Diet for Men   309

Foreword

As our obesity epidemic continues unabated, every-one is quick to point blame. A primary suspect is often the fast-food and family restaurant industry. In reality, these restaurants can end up being key players in stopping this seemingly endless battle against weight gain.

The real problem is our lack of time to prepare meals, especially meals containing the correct balance of protein, carbohydrates, and fat required to control the hormone *insulin*. Too much of this hormone is what makes us fat and keeps us fat. Fast-food and family restaurants simply present a potential solution to the problem of lack of time. If restaurant meals are organized into the right combination of protein, car-bohydrates, and fat, even people who eat out fre-quently can keep their insulin under control.

The key to slimming down and maintaining a healthy weight is keeping insulin within a range that's not too high or too low. When you manage your insulin, you continue to feel full for four to six hours and begin to burn off calories instead of storing them as fat. The best way to control your insulin is to balance protein and carbohydrates at every meal. This is the essence of my Zone Diet and of Smart-Carb eating.

This is why Tracy Jones's book can play an important role in helping you control your weight. Tracy has studied the nutritional information at fast-food and family-style restaurants, and has constructed a dietary game plan to make each meal a balanced meal.

How can eating "fatty" restaurant meals allow you to lose weight? Although fat has no direct effect on insulin, eating fat can actually *help* you access your stored body fat and burn it as energy. When you burn fat, you lose weight.

Calories for *The Smart-Carb Guide* restaurant meals are listed beside each meal. To lose weight faster, simply eat meals with fewer calories. A good rule is: Women should eat about 300 calories per meal, and men should eat about 400 calories. If these calories are properly balanced, you should not feel hungry for the next four to six hours.

This book does not propose that you eat at restaurants from morning to night, because eventually you're going to learn how to make satisfying meals yourself. But *The Smart-Carb Guide* can be a valuable resource to teach you how to make appropriate choices under any circumstance, keeping your insulin levels under control until your next meal.

My promise to you is that if you follow the guidelines and meal plans in this book, you will find it much easier to control the insulin levels in your body and lose excess body fat in the process, no matter which fast-food and family-style restaurants you visit in the future.

Barry Sears, Ph.D., author of *The Zone*

Author's Note

The Smart-Carb Guide meals use information from restaurants that was current as of the time of writing. Restaurants change their menus frequently, and may not offer some of the options listed. Differences in vendors and retesting of foods by restaurants in the future may lead to variations in the number of calories, net carbohydrates, and conformity of meals to 40-30-30 principles. Appendix A lists the formulas and criteria used to calculate the meals in this guidebook.

If you are currently taking medications, let your doctor know that your dosage may need to be adjusted after a few weeks of eating *The Smart-Carb Guide* meals. Your need for certain medications may decrease due to the tendency of 40-30-30 diets to correct hormonal imbalances and optimize health.

Medications that may need to be reduced include diuretics, insulin-stimulating drugs, and medications for lowering blood pressure. Always consult with your doctor before changing your medication dosage.

The Smart-Carb Guide to Eating Out

CHAPTER 1

• • • • • •

Can You Lose Weight by Eating Fast Food?

Yes, you can! It may be hard to believe, but eating the convenient fast-food and family restaurant meals in this book can actually help you lose weight and improve your health! Unlike the "supersized" portions most of us are used to, *The Smart-Carb Guide to Eating Out* will introduce you to balanced, moderate meals that you can enjoy at your favorite fast-food and family-style restaurants, so you can make smarter choices when eating out. If you're one of the millions of Americans who's following a sensible weight-loss plan, *The Smart-Carb Guide* can help you stay on your plan when eating out!

At this point you're probably thinking, *What's the catch?* Fad diets are common. Each one promises that you'll lose all the weight you want and feel great while eating delicious food. How is this book different? *The*

Smart-Carb Guide to Eating Out is different because there is no catch. You *can* eat foods most people think of as weight-loss no-no's—hamburgers, french fries, tacos, fried chicken, and even ice cream—and lose pounds and inches while dramatically improving your health.

There are no pills to take and no shakes to drink. You don't have to worry about counting points, calories, or carbohydrates, because we've done the counting for you! Most of the meals are inexpensive. Every meal is a treat. Best of all, you don't have to cook. All you do is go to a fast-food or family-style restaurant, open *The Smart-Carb Guide to Eating Out,* and order.

It's that simple, and it works. *The Smart-Carb Guide to Eating Out* is based on a revolutionary way of eating. The meals contain a balance of nutrients in just the right proportions. This makes it possible for you to eat your favorite foods and still lose weight, feel satisfied, and have more energy. It's what delicious, smart, healthy eating is all about.

How Does *The Smart-Carb Guide* Work?

The meals in *The Smart-Carb Guide* are based on a nutritional breakthrough called the Zone Diet, developed by Barry Sears, Ph.D. If you've heard of the Zone Diet, it may be because many movie stars, models, and athletes use it to maintain their lean, toned physiques. Or you may know someone who's used the Zone Diet to reduce their risk of diabetes, heart disease, cancer, chronic inflammation, or another major illness. The Zone Diet has often been mistakenly grouped with extreme low-carbohydrate diets. Actually, the Zone is *not* a low-carbohydrate diet. Instead, it teaches you to eat everything, including carbohydrates, in moderation. You eat a moderate amount of carbohydrates, protein, and fat in each meal—in other words, a little bit of everything. Does this sound familiar? Didn't your grandmother tell you to eat this way? Well, Grandma was right! Science has shown that eating balanced, moderate, "Smart-Carb" meals—such as those recommended by the Zone Diet—helps us stay slim and healthy throughout our lives.

Now you can follow Grandma's advice, and use science to go one step further. One of the revolutionary concepts of the Zone Diet is that there's a special balance of nutrients that helps us feel full and improves our health at the same time. It is known as 40-30-30. To make a 40-30-30 meal, you balance every 40 calories of carbohydrates with 30 calories of protein and 30 calories of fat. The meal looks like this:

Nutrient	Calories
carbohydrates	40
protein	30
fat	30

Many of today's most successful diets, including the Zone, the South Beach Diet, Sugar Busters, and the diets of many celebrity trainers, recommend meals containing this balance. *The Smart-Carb Guide* shows you how to eat these meals at your favorite restaurants. Now, instead of having to carefully count carbohydrates or calories, you can just choose one of the hundreds of balanced, moderate meals in *The Smart-Carb Guide*. The meals keep you looking great and feeling healthy and satisfied.

What's a Balanced, Moderate Meal?

With so many different ways to make meals, how do you know what a balanced, moderate meal looks like? A great example is a turkey sandwich. It's made of bread, turkey, and a little spread, like avocado or mayonnaise. The bread is mainly carbohydrates. The turkey is protein. The spread is mostly fat. If you put these ingredients together in the right proportions, a medium-size turkey sandwich can be a low-calorie meal that contains a healthy balance of carbohydrates, protein, and fat.

If it's that easy to make balanced, moderate meals, why do most of us have so much trouble losing weight? We have a hard time losing weight because the typical way we order a turkey sandwich is with chips and a soft drink. The chips and drink add extra carbohydrates and calories, throwing the meal off balance and making it more fattening. In fact, you can cut your calories *in half* simply by eating the sandwich without the chips and drink. What should you drink, then? Drink water or anything that doesn't contain calories, such as unsweetened hot tea, iced tea, or coffee. You can still have foods you like. By eating them in balance and moderation, you can satisfy your cravings whenever you want.

But wait a minute, you might be thinking. *What about the chips? What about all the other foods I like to eat, such as hamburgers, french fries, fried chicken, and ice cream? How can I eat all my favorite foods and still stay slim and healthy?*

You can eat all these foods and more—just eat them along with other foods that make your meal low in total calories and create a healthy balance of carbohydrates, protein, and fat. How do you do that? Look up the nutritional information from restaurants, examine combinations of different foods, and calculate nutritional values to create balanced meals.

Don't want to bother with all that? No problem. We've done it for you! Just order any meal in *The Smart-Carb Guide* and you'll get a balanced, low-calorie, satisfying meal that helps keep your weight down while improving your health.

The Health Benefits of Eating Balanced Meals—Even Fast-Food Meals

Thousands of people have found that eating balanced, moderate meals that follow the 40-30-30 formula developed by the Zone Diet and used by many other diets dramatically improves their health. You can experience a wide range of benefits within half an hour of eating a properly balanced meal, and continue to feel them for four to six hours. Short-term health benefits include:

+ More energy
+ Increased alertness
+ Clearer thinking
+ Better mood
+ Increased resistance to disease
+ Improved eyesight
+ Reduced carbohydrate and overall food cravings

There are also many long-term health benefits that have been reported by thousands of people. These include:

+ Easy weight loss
+ Increased muscle mass
+ Inproved athletic performance
+ Improved cholesterol levels
+ Improved triglyceride levels

+ Decreased symptoms of diabetes
+ Reduced autoimmune disease symptoms
+ Reduced arthritis symptoms
+ Less depression
+ Less anxiety
+ Fewer mood swings
+ Improved sleep patterns
+ Decreased need for sleep
+ Decreased jet lag on trips
+ Improved sexual performance
+ Decreased PMS symptoms
+ Decreased hot flashes

Why Do Smart-Carb Meals Have So Many Benefits?

There is scientific evidence that a balanced, moderate diet is how our ancestors ate. Ten thousand years ago, people ate mainly meat, fish, vegetables, fruits, and nuts. They didn't eat many foods made from grain, such as bread and rice. Grain was much harder to collect and process than other foods, so people ate less of it. By studying their bones, scientists have determined that our ancestors were strong and lean.

Today, we grow vast quantities of grain. Having developed modern ways of harvesting and processing it, we eat a great deal of bread, rice, noodles, and baked goods, all of which are grain-derived carbohydrates. While some people can eat as many

What About the "Low-Carb" Trend?

You'll notice that eating Smart-Carb meals doesn't require you to give up your favorite carbohydrates, such as bread, pasta, potatoes, and sweets, which many low-carb diets forbid. Although a very-low-carb diet may allow dieters to shed pounds quickly, the human body requires a balance of carbohydrates, protein, and fat to most effectively fuel activities and thought processes. For this reason, many low-carb dieters burn out on their plans and end up feeling less energetic and reporting other health complications.

The good news is that you don't have to cut out all or even most of your carbohydrates to lose weight. By simply balancing carbohydrates, protein, and fat while keeping your calories low, you'll experience the same weight-loss benefits that you would on a low-carbohydrate diet, without any health complications. A moderate, balanced diet allows you to eat your favorite foods in a sensible way. You can eat all the foods that make you happy, so you'll never feel deprived. It's a fun, flexible style of eating that helps you stay slim and healthy while still enjoying all the foods you love.

carbohydrates as they want and stay thin, most of us can eat only so many sweet and starchy foods before we start putting on pounds! This is because the majority of us are not suited to take in so many carbohydrates. In many ways, we're still like our ancestors of 10,000 years ago, adapted to a moderate-carbohydrate diet of vegetables, meat, nuts, and fruits. Our bodies thrive on these foods.

Let's look at an imagined recipe for a caveman meal. This is similar to what your great-great-great (and more greats) grandmother and grandfather may have eaten:

CAVEMAN DINNER (SERVES 1)

Ingredients

+ Four ounces of deer meat
+ A few handfuls of raw leaves (similar to spinach)
+ A small root (similar to a potato)
+ A handful of nuts
+ A few handfuls of blueberries

Instructions

1. Go hunt a deer. Bring it back. Clean it. Roast it.
2. Pick a bunch of leaves.

3. Dig up some roots. Roast them in the fire.
4. Collect some nuts. Remove the shells.
5. Pick some berries.

"Grandma" and "Grandpa" Caveman's dinner was moderate and balanced. If they looked at your last dinner, would they approve?

Smart-Carb Meals Versus Your Old Way of Eating

It's natural to be skeptical of an eating plan that claims a fast-food meal can be less fattening and healthier than a low-fat meal made at home, such as pasta. But if your pasta doesn't contain a healthy balance of carbohydrates, protein, and fat, and if it doesn't keep calories in check, it can actually be more fattening and less healthy than the Smart-Carb fast-food and family-style meals in this book.

But Isn't Fat Bad for You?

While nutritionists once encouraged people to avoid eating fatty foods, scientists have since learned that fat, if eaten in moderation, can actually *help* you lose weight. Fat stimulates the hormones that help you feel full. Without enough fat in your food, you may not make enough of these hormones to stay satisfied. While it's good to moderate your fat intake so you don't eat too many calories, meals containing too little fat are actually a health and weight-loss nightmare, because they leave you feeling hungry. If you've ever eaten a big bowl of low-fat pasta and felt hungry half an hour later, you understand! That's why it's important to eat enough fat in every meal— about 30 percent of the meal's calories. Does that sound like a lot? It's really just a drop in the bucket, about the amount of fat in a tablespoon or two of salad dressing. *The Smart-Carb Guide* meals contain just enough fat to keep you satisfied without adding excess calories. The result is that you lose weight without feeling hungry.

THE ULTIMATE SMART-CARB TEST: "HOW CAN I BE HUNGRY? I JUST ATE!"

Do you ever eat meals that fill you up at first but leave you hungry a short time later? Have you eaten a big bagel or muffin for breakfast and then felt famished by mid-morning? That's because bagels, muffins, and other sweet and starchy foods, when eaten alone, contain too many carbohydrates and not enough protein and fat to keep you satisfied. Eating these foods alone can also make it harder to lose weight. Three things happen when we eat foods containing too many carbohydrates without enough fat and protein:

1. We feel less energetic and more sleepy.
2. We feel hungry soon after our meal.
3. Our bodies may ultimately store more fat.

That's because carbohydrates stimulate the hormone *insulin*. High levels of insulin cause our blood sugar to drop rapidly as the sugar rushes out of our bloodstreams and into our cells. This can make us feel tired, hungry, and low-energy, and can make it difficult to lose weight. When meals contain a moderate amount of calories and carbohydrates, our body's insulin stays more stable throughout the day. This helps us feel upbeat, energetic, and satisfied. It helps our body burn fat rather than store fat, which makes weight loss easier.

"YOU ARE FEELING VERY SLEEEPYYY. . . ."
BALANCING YOUR MEALS WITH PROTEIN

Do you know the feeling of eating a lot of sugary foods at one time and experiencing a burst of energy followed by a quick drop in energy—the "sugar coma"? The same thing happens when you eat a meal that's high in starch, such as pasta. Soon after eating, you experience a drop in energy and even become sleepy—the "after-lunch coma."

Whenever a meal leaves you feeling sleepier or more sluggish than before you ate, reflect back on that meal. Did you eat mostly bread, pasta, rice, noodles, or potatoes? Did you have any protein with your meal? If your "sleepy" meal was high in carbohydrates and low in protein, make a point of adding more protein to your next meal. Chances are you'll feel less sleepy. Why? When protein is added to a meal, it helps keep your insulin level from rising too quickly.

How much protein do you need? About 30 percent of the calories in a meal. If your meal is a hamburger, that's about the amount in a medium-size hamburger patty. A good meal also contains about 40 percent carbohydrates, which is the amount in a hamburger bun. Keeping in mind that a balanced meal contains 40 percent carbohydrates, 30 percent protein, and 30 percent fat (40-30-30), let's see how some meals stack up:

MEAL	% of Calories from Carbs	% of Calories from Protein	% of Calories from Fat
Pasta with Tomato Sauce (2 cups pasta and 1 cup sauce)			
	80	15	5
2 Taco Bell Chicken Soft Tacos			
	40	29	28
Wienerschnitzel Hamburger			
	41	28	25

The pasta meal, which contains a hefty 80 percent of calories from carbohydrates and a measly 15 percent of calories from protein and 5 percent from fat, falls far short of being 40-30-30. Interestingly, despite being "fast food," the tacos and hamburger hit the mark. Because they contain a healthy balance of carbohydrates, protein, and fat calories, the tacos and the hamburger will help you stay satisfied and energized, while the pasta will tend to make you feel sleepy and low-energy.

WHAT ABOUT CALORIES?

Here are the calories for the meals:

Meal	Calories
Pasta and Tomato Sauce (2 cups pasta and one cup sauce)	480
2 Taco Bell Chicken Soft Tacos	380
Wienerschnitzel Hamburger	290

Can these numbers be correct? How can the tacos and hamburger contain fewer calories than the pasta? When a meal is balanced and moderate, like the tacos or the hamburger, it contains just enough of each nutrient without going overboard. It's moderate in carbohydrates, so it doesn't overstimulate insulin, and it contains just enough protein and fat to keep you full without adding too many calories. The result is that both of these fast-food meals are lower in calories than the pasta meal—and more satisfying.

When you choose balanced, moderate meals, whether at restaurants or at home, you'll feel full faster and for a longer time and find it easier to lose weight—the perfect recipe for a great meal!

THE DANGER OF EATING TOO MANY CALORIES AND CARBOHYDRATES

When you overeat, you may be doing damage to your health beyond increasing your appetite and making

How Do Italians Stay Healthy When They Eat So Much Pasta?

Italians traditionally eat pasta every day, yet have a lower incidence of obesity than North Americans. The traditional Italian way to eat pasta is to serve it as a small appetizer, followed by a larger main course containing fish or meat. In contrast, North Americans typically eat a large bowl of pasta that contains little or no meat. Since the traditional Italian meal is light on carbohydrates and includes protein, it's more filling than the typical North American pasta meal. A more satisfying meal means Italians are less likely to overeat and will have an easier time maintaining a healthy weight.

weight loss more difficult. You also may be making yourself sick. When your body's insulin and blood sugar fluctuate to extreme levels over long periods of time due to overeating or eating too many carbohydrates, your risk of developing type 2 diabetes, unhealthy cholesterol levels, heart disease, and cancer goes up. This is part of the reason many people experience several conditions, such as weight gain, diabetes, unhealthy cholesterol levels, and heart disease, all at the same time. These conditions all become more prevalent when the body's blood sugar and insulin are allowed to repeatedly spike to high levels over a period of years. When you eat balanced, moderate meals that keep your blood sugar and insulin in check, you reduce your risk of developing these and other chronic diseases. This makes eating well an easy and important way to increase your chances of enjoying a longer, healthier life.

What About Cholesterol and Heart Disease?

If you're concerned about cholesterol and heart disease, you may be avoiding certain foods already. The American Heart Association links saturated fats and trans-fatty acids to unhealthy cholesterol and an increased risk of heart disease. Animal foods that contain saturated fat include high-fat beef and pork, egg yolks, cheese, mayonnaise, butter, and creamy sauces and dressings. Foods high in trans-fatty acids include most margarines, fried foods, and many commercial baked products. Sound familiar? These are all commonly found on fast-food menus! Then how can a diet of fast food be healthy for people who are concerned about cholesterol and heart disease? Here are three answers to this question:

1. Choose fast-food options that are low in animal-derived saturated fats and trans-fatty acids.
2. When eating foods that contain these fats, eat smaller portions.
3. What really matters is insulin.

To reduce your intake of animal-derived saturated fats in fast food, eat meals in which the main protein comes from fish, chicken, turkey, ham, roast beef, or low-fat or nonfat milk. Also avoid mayonnaise and creamy dressings. Whenever given the choice, use olive oil rather than mayonnaise or salad dressing. To reduce your intake of trans-fatty acids, pass on fried foods and high-fat baked goods that have the words "partially hydrogenated" in the list of ingredients, which you can often find on individual restaurant websites.

If you'd still like to eat foods like hamburgers and fries, you can reduce your intake of animal-derived saturated fats and trans-fatty acids simply by eating smaller portions. Fortunately, that's exactly what *Smart-Carb Guide* meals are—smaller yet satisfying portions of your favorite foods. This makes *The Smart-Carb Guide* an excellent tool for health-conscious people who would like to enjoy their favorite foods in moderation.

What Really Matters?

Talking about saturated fat raises an interesting question. There is a group of people who eat butter, cream, cheese, beef, or pork with almost every meal—yet have far lower rates of obesity, diabetes, and heart disease than North Americans. These people are the French. Traditional French food uses animal fats as its main fat source. French people, as well as many other Europeans, put real cream in their cereal, cook with plenty of butter, and eat eggs, cheese, and high-fat meats regularly. Why are these people able to live relatively healthy lives with comparatively low rates of heart disease while North Americans, many of whom have long since given up eating butter, cream, and whole eggs, are caught in an escalating epidemic of heart disease, obesity, diabetes, and cancer? The answer may lie in *how* the French eat their meals.

Traditional French meals are small, high in fat, and moderate in carbohydrates and protein. Small meals that balance carbohydrates with protein help control insulin. When insulin is kept under control, people are not as hungry and feel satisfied eating smaller portions. Also, lower insulin levels help the body burn fat rather than storing fat. The moderate portion size and balance in French cuisine helps the French stay thin, and that may be a reason they have lower rates of diabetes and heart disease.

So eating with balance and moderation may be important for maintaining healthy cholesterol levels and reducing your risk of heart disease. While it's important to include a variety of healthy foods in your diet, keep in mind the possibility that *how* you eat can also greatly affect your health. If this is true, then eating small portions of foods that contain animal-derived saturated fat, such as cheeseburgers, may not be quite as bad for us as we imagine. And eating large, unbalanced meals made from low-fat, high-carbohydrate foods, such as pasta, may be worse for us than we imagine.

How to Use *The Smart-Carb Guide* with Your Weight-Loss Plan

One of the best features of *The Smart-Carb Guide* is that you can fit the restaurant meals listed in the book into your own weight-loss plan. Now you have an easy way to stay on your diet, even when eating out with friends and family, grabbing meals on the run, and indulging in your favorite fast-food treats.

THE ZONE

All the meals in *The Smart-Carb Guide* are designed to work with the Zone Diet because they've been formulated based on the 40-30-30 principles introduced by Barry Sears, Ph.D., in *The Zone* (ReganBooks, 1995). You can substitute a Smart-Carb meal for any Zone meal. The sections Smart-Carb Snacks and Smart-Carb Salads (pages 32 and 40) are tools you can use to help you follow the Zone Diet at home.

THE SOUTH BEACH DIET

The Smart-Carb Guide meals can be used during Phase 3 of the South Beach Diet, the maintenance phase that allows you the most freedom in carbohydrate choices. *The Smart-Carb Guide* is ideal for people who want to treat themselves to restaurant meals while still maintaining a healthy weight and suppressing carbohydrate cravings. Smart-Carb Salads (page 40) and Smart-Carb Snacks (page 32) can also be eaten during Phase 2 of the South Beach Diet. *The Smart-Carb Guide* is not recommended for use with Phase 1 of the South Beach Diet, during which carbohydrate choices are more limited.*

*The recommendation to use *The Smart-Carb Guide to Eating Out* with the South Beach Diet is solely the opinion of this author and is based on this author's interpretation of descriptions given in *The South Beach Diet*. It is not meant to imply endorsement of this book by the author of *The South Beach Diet* or any affiliated company or party.

OTHER 40-30-30 DIETS

Smart-Carb Guide meals are based on 40-30-30 principles and can be used with other 40-30-30 eating plans, including The Formula and many diets used by celebrity trainers. For a description of how the meals were calculated, please see Appendix A.

DOES THE SMART-CARB GUIDE WORK WITH THE ATKINS DIET?

If you are on the Atkins Diet or another low-carbohydrate diet that recommends a certain number of net carbohydrates per day, you can use the information on net carbohydrates listed beside each meal to select meals that allow you to stay within your diet's daily carbohydrate limits.

Getting Started Eating Smart-Carb Meals

Since they're balanced and low in calories, *Smart-Carb Guide* meals are the perfect way to eat out. They'll make you feel more upbeat and energetic and help you lose weight—even when you're eating at fast-food and family-style restaurants. Once you experience how great you'll look and feel when eating the balanced, moderate meals in this book, you'll want to learn how to make similar meals at home. A great way to begin making meals at home is to follow the instructions for making Smart-Carb Salads (page 40), which can be created either at salad bars or from ingredients in your kitchen. Whether you eat at home or at restaurants, so long as your meals contain a healthy balance of carbohydrates, protein, and fat, and are low in calories, you'll feel healthy, satisfied, and full of energy.

Are you ready to eat out the Smart-Carb way?

CHAPTER 2

How to Lose Weight Eating Smart-Carb Meals

Losing weight with *The Smart-Carb Guide* is easy. Whether you're on a weight-loss plan already or are looking for an easy way to slim down, you'll be able to use the meals in this book to help lose weight and stay satisfied. You can choose to eat Smart-Carb meals for breakfast, lunch, or dinner—or for all of your meals. The 7-Day Quick-Start Diet will help you lose weight quickly and easily with preplanned menus for each day. There are tips on how to make your own Smart-Carb Salads and snacks that can be added to your weight-loss program or used with the 7-Day Quick-Start Diet. Here are some different ways you can use *The Smart-Carb Guide to Eating Out* to lose weight:

✦ **Enjoy Smart-Carb Meals at Your Favorite Restaurants.** Simply use the menus in chapters 3 and 4 to lose weight while eating delicious meals at your favorite restaurants.

✦ **Lose Weight Fast with the 7-Day Quick-Start Diet.** Jump-start your weight loss by following the 7-Day Quick-Start Diet. Just tear out the meal cards in the back of this book to get on the fast track to losing weight and staying healthy.

✦ **Eat Healthier at Fast-Food and Family Restaurants.** Even if you eat fast food infrequently, you can use *The Smart-Carb Guide to Eating Out* to make healthier choices that will help you maintain a healthy weight and high energy level.

✦ **Get Back on Track After a Period of Overindulging.** We all get into the habit of eating too much at times, especially around holidays. Eating the balanced, moderate meals listed in *The Smart-Carb Guide* will help you break overeating habits quickly and will get you back to eating healthy portions.

✦ **Experience Eating Balanced, Moderate Meals.** Use *Smart-Carb Guide* meals to remind yourself what a good meal feels like—it leaves you satisfied rather than overly full, and energetic rather than sleepy. Once you've experienced the benefits of eating Smart-Carb restaurant meals, you'll want to make your own balanced, satisfying meals at home. You can start right away by following the easy instructions for making Smart-Carb Salads (page 40).

The *Smart-Carb Guide* Menus

Meals in *The Smart-Carb Guide* are separated into sections for women (chapter 3) and for men (chapter 4). They're divided this way because men typically need a little more food than women to maintain their health and energy. Women can order a meal from the men's section, eat three-fourths of it, and save the rest for a snack. Men can order a meal from the women's section and make it more filling by eating it with a Smart-Carb Snack (page 32). To lose weight more quickly, eat one of the lower-calorie meals or substitute Smart-Carb Salads for some of the restaurant meals (page 40).

The Smart-Carb Guide provides a separate menu for each restaurant. Meals on the menus tell you exactly what to eat. There are a variety of meals to choose from, all of which are moderate and balanced, so you can order any meal you like. If a restaurant serves breakfast, there will usually be two menus: one for breakfast, and one that includes both lunch and dinner. The menus in this book list meals just like menus at a restaurant. Instead of prices, to the right of each meal are the calories and net carbohydrates.

WHY ARE CALORIES AND NET CARBOHYDRATES LISTED?

Calories and net carbohydrates (total carbohydrates minus fiber) are provided simply for your reference and to help integrate *Smart-Carb Guide* meals into other diet plans that have particular requirements. You don't need to consider calories and net carbohydrates when choosing your meals. **All the meals are designed to be balanced and moderate to help you lose weight.** Feel free to ignore calories and net carbohydrates and order any meal you like.

ORDERING MEALS FROM THE MENUS

When ordering meals from *The Smart-Carb Guide*, eat everything that's listed with a meal. Don't add anything extra, or the meal won't be balanced. For example, this is how *The Smart-Carb Guide* lists an A&W Hamburger:

MEAL	CALORIES	NET CARBS
Hamburger	460	36

Since fries and a soda aren't listed with the meal, eat just the hamburger with water or an unsweetened drink. Are you ever allowed to eat fries? Sure! Just order a meal that includes fries, like this McDonald's meal:

Meal	Calories	Net Carbs
Chicken McGrill Sandwich (no bun)	450	31
Small Fries 1 package ketchup		

Notice that the meal tells you to eat the chicken sandwich *without the bread*. This way, you get to eat fries while still eating a meal that contains the right amount of total calories and carbohydrates.

As you become more familiar with the menus, you may notice that some meals look alike but are actually slightly different. These variations are included to give you more options for ordering meals the way you like them.

FOLLOWING THE MEAL DIRECTIONS

+ **Splitting Meals.** Some meals, particularly at the family restaurants, are made up of menu items that you should only eat half of per meal. These meals can be split with another person, such as a friend who eats with you at the restaurant, or if you order the meal for yourself, you can eat half of it and save the rest for a later meal. Some of these splittable meals have a How to Order instruction that tells you what to order to serve two.

✦ **How to Order.** Some meals include a section called How to Order. This is a script, using the restaurant's own lingo, that you can read to your server so that they understand how to prepare your food and they know which condiments to bring to you.

Should I Order from the Low-Carb Menus at Restaurants?

Many restaurants now offer low-carbohydrate alternatives to their regular meals. These meals are typically high in protein and fat and very low in carbohydrates—such as a large hamburger with mayonnaise but without a bun. Meals such as these, while appropriate for people on very-low-carbohydrate diets, don't match the Smart-Carb criteria for a balanced meal. The low-carb options contain too much protein and fat and not enough carbohydrates. The meals chosen for *The Smart-Carb Guide* always include a moderate amount of all three major nutrients: carbohydrates, protein, and fat. An example of a Smart-Carb meal would be a medium-size hamburger *with* the bun but without mayonnaise. Since the only difference between the typical Smart-Carb hamburger and a regular hamburger is that you ask your server to hold the mayo, Smart-Carb meals start out as regular meals (rather than low-carb versions) and are modified as needed.

The 7-Day Quick-Start Diet

To jump-start your weight loss with simple pre-planned menus, try the 7-Day Quick-Start Diet. The directions are listed below, and you can find the women's and men's menus listed on cards in the back of the book. Tear out the cards and take them with you when you go to restaurants and order your meals.

BENEFITS OF THE 7-DAY QUICK-START DIET

✦ **Losing Weight.** The 7-Day Quick-Start Diet is a great way to begin a balanced, moderate eating program that will improve your health while helping you lose weight. In the first week, you can lose up to five pounds. After that, most people continue to lose one to two pounds a week. In case you're wondering whether this is fast or slow, one to two pounds per week is the maximum healthy weight loss. When people go on "crash diets" and lose weight faster than this, they're losing fluids and muscle mass rather than fat. Losing weight at the healthy rate is an indication that you're losing fat rather than muscle.

Beware of the Scale!

Don't let the number on the scale fool you. If you gain muscle while losing fat (the best of both worlds), the two may cancel each other out so that your weight on the scale stays the same. So the weight on the scale won't always tell you whether or not you're losing fat. How do you know for sure if you're losing fat? Should you go out and buy a body caliper or do a laboratory test to find out your body fat composition? Nope. Just do a "pants test." If your pants fit more loosely than before, congratulations, you're losing fat!

In fact, if you exercise regularly while following the Smart-Carb plan, you're likely to increase your muscle mass while losing fat.

+ **Sizing Up Portions.** Have you ever wondered how much food you really need to stay satisfied? When you follow the 7-Day Quick-Start Diet, you'll get a crash course on eating the right portion sizes to lose weight and stay healthy. It's not a typical course, where you study and take tests. In this course, all you do is—you guessed it—eat! Just order meals from the preprinted cards, eat, and see how you feel. At the end of the week, see how much weight you've lost and decide whether you enjoy eating moderate, balanced meals. Decide if you'd like to follow this healthy way of eating in the future by making moderate, balanced meals at home. Does learning to eat right get any more fun or easier than that? *Bon appétit!*

How to Follow the 7-Day Quick-Start Diet

Meals on the 7-Day Quick-Start Diet are organized by restaurant. For example, Day 1 is Arby's day. They are just listed this way for convenience—all of the meals from all of the restaurants are interchangeable. So on the same day, you can eat at McDonald's for breakfast, Subway for lunch, and Wendy's for dinner. And you don't have to stop the diet after seven days! Simply substitute other meals from the Smart-Carb menus in the book for the 7-Day Diet meals. And you can always substitute a Smart-Carb Salad (page 40), made at home or at a salad bar, for any meal on the plan.

Directions for following the 7-Day Quick-Start Diet are simple:

1. Eat meals exactly as they're written on the cards.

2. Eat 3 meals and 2 snacks per day.
3. Don't drink anything sweet.
4. Get your vitamins.

Smart-Carb Snacks

Eating the Smart-Carb way includes eating delicious, filling snacks. To feel satisfied and energetic throughout the day, eat two snacks: one in the late afternoon and one before going to bed. Eating a small Smart-Carb Snack before bed actually helps balance your hormones, aiding weight loss and sleep.

If you're physically active, you can eat one or two extra snacks on the days you exercise—which is a good reason to work out! Choose snacks you enjoy and that are convenient, satisfying, and economical.

WHAT'S A SMART-CARB SNACK?

Smart-Carbs Snacks are snacks that have a healthy balance of carbohydrates and protein, and contain about 100 calories. The snacks are the same for women and men. Easy, affordable, wholesome Smart-Carb Snacks can be made using the following foods:

+ Nuts
+ Protein and fruit
+ Milk or yogurt

NUTS

A handful of nuts makes a perfect Smart-Carb Snack! The amount of nuts that fits in most people's closed fist (with no nuts showing) is about two tablespoons. This is the right amount for a snack. It's enough to give you energy but is still low in calories. Most nuts contain healthy fats that are good for your heart, as well as Vitamin E, which is good for your skin.

You can purchase any type of nuts for your Smart-Carb Snacks, including almonds, pistachios, cashews, pecans, peanuts, and macadamia nuts. You can eat the nuts whole, chopped, or sliced. Most nuts can be eaten either raw or roasted, but some people experience stomach upset when eating certain nuts raw, especially cashews and pistachios. To be safe, buy cashews, pistachios, and other nuts that you may be sensitive to roasted rather than raw. Nuts can be either dry-roasted or oil-roasted; dry-roasted nuts are a bit lower in calories, but the difference is small. Both salted and unsalted nuts are fine, though unsalted nuts are recommended if you'd like to cut down on sodium.

Nuts are a perfect lightweight, go-anywhere food. Keep them with you at work or in the trunk of your car, and you'll always have a pick-me-up on hand. When you work out, take two handfuls of nuts with you in a small container or plastic bag. Eat a handful about 20 minutes before exercising and another

Are You a Nut-a-holic?

Most people find that salted nuts are easier to
overeat than unsalted nuts, so nut-a-holics
may want to choose the unsalted kind. If you
tend to eat too many nuts once you start,
here's a great trick: Keep a package of nuts in
the trunk of your car—*not* in the passenger
compartment, where you might be tempted to
munch on them while in traffic. Grab a handful
of nuts from your trunk whenever you need a
quick snack.

Another trick that will ensure that you get
the right amount of nuts for your snack is to
store them in small 2-ounce plastic salsa and
salad-dressing containers, available at take-out
restaurants and salad bars. Check the bottom
of the containers to make sure they say "2 oz."
Each 2-ounce container holds enough nuts for
two snacks. For one snack, fill the container
halfway. The containers fit in your pocket or
purse, and they make ideal carrying cases for
snacks when you're exercising or away from
home.

handful within 20 minutes afterward. Eating balanced snacks like nuts before and after you exercise improves athletic performance, helping you get the most out of your workout.

PROTEIN AND FRUIT

Protein and fruit, eaten together, is a satisfying snack that makes good use of leftovers. When meat and fruit are eaten together, they're much more filling than either one eaten alone. The protein in meat balances the carbohydrates in the fruit, keeping you full longer. When restaurant meals contain too much meat or other protein, you can take the extra protein home and combine it with fruit to make healthy, economical snacks. The *Smart-Carb Guide* menus tell you how many snacks you can make from any protein that's left over after you finish your meal. To make a protein and fruit snack, choose one protein and one fruit from table 2.1.

TABLE 2.1
Protein and Fruit for Snacks*

Protein	Fruit
¼ cup cottage cheese	⅓ medium apple (or ½ small apple)

*Adapted from *The Zone* (Barry Sears, Ph.D., 1995).

Protein	Fruit
¾ ounce cheese	½ medium orange (or 1 small orange)
¼ cup grated cheese	1 large apricot
1 ounce turkey	1 small to medium plum
1 ounce chicken	½ large peach
1 ounce fish	1 cup strawberries
1 ounce beef	⅓ cup grapes
1 ounce ham	⅓ medium pear
2 Tbsp. soy nuts	⅓ medium banana

The two examples on the next page show you how to combine protein and fruit from table 2.1 to make snacks. Notice that the proteins and fruits are interchangeable—you can combine any protein with any fruit. Create your own protein-and-fruit snack by filling in the blank spaces on the chart on the next page.

Smart-Carb Tip: Two Thumbs Up!

An ounce of meat, fish, or cheese is about the size of your two thumbs put together.

Protein and Fruit Snack #1

Food	Choice
1 Protein	1 ounce turkey
1 Fruit	½ medium orange

Protein and Fruit Snack #2

Food	Choice
1 Protein	¾ ounce cheese
1 Fruit	½ small apple

Make Your Own Protein and Fruit Snack!

Food	Your Choice
1 Protein	
1 Fruit	

MILK OR YOGURT

Milk or plain yogurt provides the perfect balance of protein and carbohydrates. For a Smart-Carb Snack, have ¾ cup of milk or yogurt. When buying yogurt, choose the *plain* kind, as the flavored varieties contain sweeteners that add extra carbohydrates. You can use milk or yogurt with any fat content: whole, reduced-fat, low-fat, or nonfat (skim).

The following recipe for Hot Vanilla Milk was given to me by cookbook author Debbie Puente (www.CremeBrulee.com). It makes a soothing bed-time snack.

HOT VANILLA MILK

¾ cup milk
¼ tsp. vanilla extract

Heat the milk just until hot. Do not allow to boil. Add vanilla. Stir and enjoy!

What Can I Drink?

Drink a glass of water or other unsweetened drink with your meals, such as unsweetened sparkling water, hot tea, iced tea, or coffee. For a refreshing drink, squeeze the juice from a small lemon or lime wedge into a glass of plain or sparkling water.

Smart-Carb meals don't include regular soft drinks, since soft drinks add extra carbohydrates and can cause your blood sugar and insulin levels to rise rapidly. Over time, this may jeopardize your health and prevent you from losing weight. Fruit juices, although often perceived as being healthy, contain about as many carbohydrates as soft drinks and may also cause a rapid rise in blood sugar and insulin levels. While they're not recommended, diet beverages and calorie-free sweeteners such as Splenda,

Sweet'N Low, and Equal are allowed on the Smart-Carb plan.

GETTING YOUR VITAMINS

When following the 7-Day Quick-Start Diet or eating at fast-food restaurants frequently, it's important to supplement your diet with foods that are high in vitamins, minerals, and fiber. A good way to ensure that you get these nutrients is to eat at least one salad a day, especially salads containing dark green leafy vegetables. These include dark green romaine, green leaf, and red leaf lettuce, baby greens, and spinach. Many restaurants now offer salads containing a mix of these and lighter lettuces.

You can give your health an even bigger boost by eating a Smart-Carb Salad (page 40) for at least one of your meals. Another great option is simply to add green leafy vegetables to your meals and snacks. Both raw and cooked greens are excellent sources of nutrients, contain very few calories and carbohydrates, and can actually help you lose weight by helping you stay full. On the Smart-Carb plan, you can eat as much of them as you like.

To make a simple salad, place one to two oversized handfuls of dark green lettuce, spinach, or baby greens in a large bowl. Mix with ½ Tbsp. vinegar or lemon juice and a little salt, pepper, garlic, and mustard to taste. (See more about salads on p. 40.)

To prepare cooked greens, steam or boil leafy greens such as collard greens, kale, chard, turnip greens, bok choy, and spinach (be sure to wash them well before cooking). Flavor with any combination of salt, pepper, lemon juice, hot sauce, vinegar, and garlic.

Smart-Carb Salads

Enjoying a salad every day will provide you with vitamins, minerals, and fiber that will help you feel great and boost your health. If prepared the right way, a salad can be a hearty, satisfying meal. Smart-Carb Salads are complete meals that you can eat *in place of* any fast-food or family-style meal in *The Smart-Carb Guide.* You can make a Smart-Carb Salad anywhere that has a salad bar—at restaurants, supermarkets, take-out salad bars, and even pizza

---

Smart-Carb Salad Ingredients
1. Lettuce
2. Other vegetables
3. Protein
4. Dressing
5. Fruit

---

parlors. You can also make Smart-Carb Salads at home, using ingredients you may already have in your refrigerator.

1. **Lettuce:** 2 cups of dark green lettuce, spinach, or baby greens.
2. **Other Vegetables:** 1–2 cups of your favorite vegetables, except for beans and corn (baby corn ears are okay). If you'd like to add beans and corn to your salad, see the sidebar on beans and corn on page 45.
3. **Protein:** Include some protein with your salad to balance the carbohydrates and help keep you full. Here are the amounts to use for chicken, tuna, cottage cheese, soybeans, and tofu:

> **Chicken or tuna:**
> Women: ½ cup
> Men: ⅔ cup
>
> **Cottage cheese***¹
> Women: ¼ cup
> Men: 1 cup

---

*Cottage cheese, soybeans, and tofu also contain carbohydrates. When eating them, eat half as much fruit in your salad (see page 44).

How Much Is a Cup?

You can use your hands to estimate the size of
one cup. Cup both of your hands together in
front of you as though you were drinking
water from a faucet. The amount of food that
would fit in your hands is about one cup.
When you estimate cups of food, you can use
your cupped hands as a visual guide. To estimate ½ cup, just take half of what would fit
in your hands. Estimate similarly for ⅓ cup,
⅔ cup, and ¾ cup.

Soybeans (edamame), shelled:*
Women: ¾ cup
Men: 1 cup

Tofu (firm 1-inch cubes):†
Women: 9 cubes
Men: 12 cubes

---

*Cottage cheese, soybeans, and tofu also contain carbohydrates.
When eating them, eat half as much fruit in your salad (see
page 44).
†Edamame (shelled green soybeans) and tofu contain fat. When
adding them to your salad, use vinegar instead of olive oil or
salad dressing.

4. **Dressing:** You can either add your own olive oil and vinegar to your salad or use a prepared salad dressing such as ranch, Caesar, Italian, or blue cheese. You need to add fat to your salad so you'll stay full, so choose a regular salad dressing rather than a low-fat variety. Use ½ to 1 tablespoon of vinegar when adding your own olive oil and vinegar to your salad. (See table 2.2 for olive oil measurements.) When taking a salad to go, keep the salad dressing (or oil and vinegar) separate from your salad. Add it to the salad just before eating. This prevents the acid in the dressing from wilting the lettuce.

5. **Fruit:** You can choose fruit from the salad bar, or if you're at a supermarket, you can save

How Much Is a Tablespoon?

You can use your fingers to estimate a tablespoon. Touch the tips of your thumb and first finger together to make a circle. This is the hand gesture people make when saying "A-OK!" The circle your fingers make holds about one tablespoon. Half of the circle holds about one-half tablespoon.

money by choosing fruit from the produce section. Pick one fruit from table 2.3 to eat with your salad.

TABLE 2.2
Dressing Portions for Smart-Carb Salads

	Women	Men
Olive oil	1/2 Tbsp.	1 Tbsp.
Salad dressing	1 Tbsp.	2 Tbsp.

TABLE 2.3
Fruit Portions for Smart-Carb Salads

Women	Men
1 small apple (or ½ medium apple)	1 medium apple
1 medium orange	1 large orange (or 2 small oranges)
½ medium pear	1 medium pear
1 small banana	1 medium banana
1 medium peach	2 small peaches
1 small nectarine	1 medium-to-large nectarine

Beans and Corn

If you'd like, you can add either beans or corn to your salad. Because beans and corn add extra carbohydrates, if you choose to eat them, don't add fruit. You can use beans, corn, or a combination of the two. Add these total amounts to your salad:

Women: 1/3 cup
Men: 1/2 cup

Women	Men
2 large apricots	3 large apricots
1 large plum	2 medium plums
1 cup honeydew	1 3/4 cups honeydew
1 1/4 cups cantaloupe	2 cups cantaloupe
1/2 cup grapes	3/4 cup grapes
1 1/4 cups strawberries	2 1/2 cups strawberries

Eating Extra Food

Men and women who are physically active or who have an extra-large build may need to eat more food.

If you exercise strenuously several times a week or are significantly heavier or taller than average, add extra food during the day.

The best times to eat extra food are 1) in the morning, since food eaten earlier in the day is burned off more easily, and 2) twenty minutes before and after you exercise. If you're active, one way to add extra food is simply to eat a snack twenty minutes before and twenty minutes after you work out or do a strenuous activity. This gives your body extra fuel when you need it and helps make your workout more effective. If your exercise falls close to a mealtime, you can eat a snack before exercising, then follow your workout with a meal. For instance, you might eat a snack soon after waking up, then go for a walk or run, then eat breakfast soon afterward.

The following are healthy ways to eat extra food on the Smart-Carb plan.

Women
1. Eat 1–3 extra Smart-Carb Snacks per day, or
2. Eat a men's meal for one or more of your meals.

Men
1. Eat 1–3 extra Smart-Carb Snacks per day, or
2. Eat a Jumbo Meal, listed at the end of the men's menu, for one or more of your meals.

What if I Still Feel Hungry?

Smart-Carb meals are balanced to ensure that your body receives the nutrients it needs to keep you energized and satisfied for four to six hours. However, in some cases, you may still feel hungry between Smart-Carb meals. There are several reasons why you may be feeling hungry.

+ **The Smart-Carb portion sizes are smaller than you're used to.** Eating less food may make you think that you should be feeling hungry. Many of us, especially in North America, are used to eating a lot of food at every meal. Portion sizes in most restaurants have doubled since the 1950s. *The Smart-Carb Guide* will help you become accustomed to the more moderate portions people ate fifty years ago, at a time when North Americans were far less prone to obesity.

+ **Your food hasn't settled yet.** Sometimes you may feel hungry right after eating, especially if you ate quickly. Wait twenty minutes, and then consider whether your meal has filled you up.

+ **You skipped your last meal.** Be sure to eat three evenly spaced meals and two snacks per day. If you skip meals, you will be hungry. If you want Smart-Carb meals to satisfy you, you must eat regularly.

✦ **You added extra carbohydrates to your last meal.** If you add a soft drink or any extra carbohydrates to your meal, you may feel hungry soon after eating. The extra carbohydrates cause your insulin level to shoot up, making you more likely to feel hungry.

✦ **You're used to eating at a certain time.** If you always have doughnuts at 10 A.M., then when 10 A.M. rolls around, your body will crave doughnuts. Resist the urge to carbo-load. Your body will quickly retrain itself to feel comfortable eating on whatever schedule you set.

✦ **There were not enough calories in your last meal.** This may happen if you engage in intense physical work or exercise, or if you have a larger build. If you fit into one of these categories, consider eating the higher-calorie meals listed toward the end of each menu. Also, see Eating Extra Food (page 45).

✦ **You may be tired or anxious.** Fatigue and anxiety can lead to "stress eating." If you're tired, you'll benefit from getting some rest. If you're anxious, ask yourself what you can do— aside from eating—to solve the problem that's making you anxious. Often, simply acknowledging a problem is enough to get you focused on solving it, and that may reduce your desire to eat.

+ **You may be accustomed to overeating.** Most people overeat at one time or another, for a variety of reasons. Sometimes food just looks good and is hard to resist. Other times we feel nervous, depressed, stressed, bored, or lonely. Whatever the reason, overeating, just like eating too many carbohydrates, causes our bodies to release a surge of insulin. When you're on a balanced, moderate diet, the need to overeat, while still present at times, decreases, because your meals control the insulin in your body. By keeping your insulin levels balanced throughout the day, the meals help you feel full and help reduce carbohydrate cravings. Though you may still overeat at times, if you make balanced, moderate eating a habit, you'll overeat far less often than before.

If you'd like to reduce your tendency to overeat, consider following the 7-Day Quick-Start Diet (see the tear-out cards in the back of the book). It will help you get into the habit of eating small, balanced meals on a regular schedule without feeling hungry.

Putting a Lid on Emotional Overeating

Many people feel that if they could only stop overeating when they feel anxious or sad, they'd never have to worry about food or weight gain again. Life would be so much simpler and happier. Exercise physiologist and *The Oprah Winfrey Show* guest Bob Greene says that when you overeat for emotional reasons, what you're really seeking is love. You crave unconditional acceptance. You yearn for the kind of love that tells you everything's okay, that you really didn't mess up, that no one can make you feel bad, that you will have all the things you want, and that everything will be all right. Just imagine what your life would be like if you always felt completely secure, at ease, and happy! Some people seem to feel this way, or close to it, whenever they want. Would you like to?

One way to look at this is that all it takes for any of us to feel this way is a single decision not to let things make us unhappy. This may sound unrealistic and maybe even counterproductive. After all, don't people need to feel bad? Isn't that a part of how we improve ourselves?

Exactly! When something begins to bother us, we can use it as an opportunity to immediately find a solution to the problem. Alternatively, we can set the problem aside for a while, decide to work on it later, and make our sense of happiness our immediate, number-one priority. Or we can do what so many of us do and delay both of these options, sliding into a sense of negativity and a belief that we are helpless to change things. And yet, strangely, all it takes to change our state of mind into a secure, confident one is the *decision* to feel good.

Believe that you deserve only the best. Believe that you are the star in the show of your life. When nothing has the power to make you unhappy, you won't need to overeat or use other coping mechanisms to turn down the volume of your desires. Your desires are important and fundamental to you. Listen to them. They will immediately point you toward the road to happiness. But you must make a *daily decision* not to let anything interfere with the belief that you can, and deserve, to have the life you want.

The Smart-Carb Guide was written as an entry point to a better life, a guidebook to help

(continued)

you in your search for health and happiness. Its goal is to open the door to balanced, moderate eating, a lifestyle that improves your well-being while making it easy, often effortless, to lose weight by allowing you to feel full while eating less. It's an exciting tool that's now in your hands. Use it to pave the way to fantastic health and a long, active, joyous life!

Tips for Improving Weight Loss

These surefire tips will help you lose weight even faster and more easily when eating the Smart-Carb way:

1. **Exercise.** Engage in the types of exercise activities that you like. Any form of exercise is great: walking (even walking around the mall), bike riding, weight lifting, swimming, shooting hoops, even a night dancing on the town. Can't afford a StairMaster? Try running up and down the stairs in your home or office building. Prefer to watch your favorite TV show? March in place in front of your TV and do jumping jacks during commercials! Any

exercise you choose to do is a gift to your body. So, are you ready to treat yourself?

2. **Eat Dinner Early.** Start dinner at about 5 P.M. You'll be amazed at how much easier weight loss becomes with this one change. The purpose of eating a late-afternoon snack is to hold you over until dinner, so if you eat dinner early, you can skip your afternoon snack. Always eat your bedtime snack, however, as it helps balance your metabolism.

3. **Make Dinner a Smart-Carb Salad.** Eat a Smart-Carb Salad (page 40) or another salad listed in the book for dinner. Eating vegetables and fruits rather than starches at night helps speed up weight loss.

So, are you ready to begin eating easy, delicious Smart-Carb meals? Then pull up a chair—or pull up to the drive-thru window—and enjoy!

CHAPTER 3

· · · · · ·

Smart-Carb
Women's Meals

A&W Women   Lunch/Dinner

MEAL	CALORIES	NET CARBS
2 Chicken Strips	333	20
With ½ BBQ Sauce	353	24
With ½ Sweet-and-Sour Sauce	355	26
¾ Deluxe Hamburger (no dressing)	330	25
With ketchup and mustard	360	29
With dressing	375	27
¾ Hamburger	345	27

MEAL	CALORIES	NET CARBS
¾ Deluxe Cheeseburger (no dressing)	360	27
¾ Cheeseburger	375	30

APPLEBEE'S Women   Lunch/Dinner

MEAL	CALORIES	NET CARBS
Grilled Tilapia with Mango Salsa	348	34

1½ soup spoons of Italian, Caesar, Blue Cheese, or Ranch Dressing on the meal (order it on the side with a soup spoon)

Eat ⅔ of the fish (save the rest for a snack). Eat all the rice and vegetables. You can use the lemon if you like.

Snacks: Extra fish = 1 Protein

Teriyaki Shrimp Skewers	311	34

1½ Soup Spoons of Italian, Caesar, Blue Cheese, or Ranch Dressing on the meal (order dressing on the side with a soup spoon)

Don't use the teriyaki dipping sauce. Eat just 6 shrimp (save the rest for snacks). Eat all of the rice and vegetables. You can use the lemon if you like.

Snacks: 2 shrimp = 1 Protein

Half-size Chicken
Caesar Salad   308   26

(chicken on the side, no Parmesan, no croutons, no dressing, no garlic toast)

1 soup spoon of Caesar, Ranch, Blue Cheese, or Italian Dressing (order dressing on the side with a soup spoon)

1 lemon wedge (order it on the side)

½ Chocolate Raspberry Layer Cake

Remove ⅓ of the chicken (an amount slightly larger than 2 thumbs put together). This can be saved for a snack. To the lettuce, add 1 soup spoon of dressing, the juice from the lemon wedge, and black pepper to taste. Mix with your fork. Put the remaining ⅔ of the chicken back on the salad.

Don't forget to eat ½ piece of Chocolate Raspberry Layer cake for dessert.

Snacks: Extra Chicken = 1 Protein

MEAL	CALORIES	NET CARBS
Half-Size Chicken Caesar Salad	308	21

(chicken on the side, no Parmesan, no croutons, no dressing, no garlic toast)

1 soup spoon of Caesar, Ranch, Blue Cheese, or Italian Dressing (order dressing on the side with a soup spoon)

1 lemon wedge (order it on the side)

½ piece of Berry Lemon Cheesecake

Remove ⅓ of the chicken (an amount slightly larger than 2 thumbs put together). This can be saved for a snack. To the lettuce, add 1 soup spoon of dressing, the juice from the lemon wedge, and black pepper to taste. Mix with your fork. Put the remaining ⅔ of the chicken back on the salad.

Don't forget to eat ½ piece of Cheesecake for dessert.

With ⅔ piece of Cheesecake	346	27
With ¾ piece of Cheesecake	365	30

Snacks: Extra Chicken = 1 Protein

MEAL	CALORIES	NET CARBS

Sizzling Chicken Skillet   292   30

1 Soup Spoon of Ranch, Blue Cheese, Caesar, or Italian Dressing on the meal (order dressing on the side with a soup spoon)

Don't eat the Ranch Dressing that comes with the meal. Remove the 2 largest pieces of chicken (save for a snack). Eat just 2 pre-sliced tortilla pieces, the remaining chicken, and the vegetables. Add 1 soup spoon of the salad dressing that *you* ordered on the side (*not* the Ranch Dressing that comes with the meal). Have as much of the salsa and lemon as you like.

Snacks: Extra chicken = 1 Protein

**Half-Size Chicken
Caesar Salad**   299   17

(chicken on the side, no Parmesan, no dressing, no garlic toast)

1 soup spoon of Caesar, Ranch, Blue Cheese, or Italian Dressing (order dressing on the side with a soup spoon)

1 lemon wedge (order it on the side)

Remove ⅓ of the chicken (an amount
slightly larger than 2 thumbs put together).
To the lettuce, add 1 soup spoon of dressing,
the juice from the lemon wedge, and
black pepper to taste. Mix with your fork.
Add the remaining ⅔ of the chicken to
the salad.

Snacks: Extra Chicken = 1 Protein

ARBY'S Women   Lunch/Dinner

Condiments:
+ Ketchup: up to ½ packet

MEAL	CALORIES	NET CARBS
Regular Roast Beef Sandwich	350	32
Hot Ham & Cheese Sandwich	300	34
Asian Sesame Salad (no noodles, no almonds)	360	28
Asian Sesame Dressing (all)		

MEAL	CALORIES	NET CARBS
Asian Sesame Salad with Noodles (no almonds)	336	28

½ Asian Sesame Dressing
Save the almonds for a snack.

MEAL	CALORIES	NET CARBS
¾ French Dip Sub (without Au Jus Sauce)	330	30
With Au Jus Sauce	334	31
¾ Grilled Chicken Deluxe Sandwich (with everything)	308	28

AU BON PAIN   Women   Breakfast

Tips:

+ Bagel sandwiches were calculated on plain bagels. You can substitute other varieties, but calories and net carbohydrates may vary slightly.

Meal	Calories	Net Carbs
Eggs with Roasted Peppers	285	20
1 Piece Artisan Multigrain Bread		
Eggs with ½ Piece Cheddar Cheese	303	30
Medium Apple With ½ Piece Mozzarella Cheese	303	31
1 Egg with Brie Cheese	350	30
½ Bagel		
½ Eggs with Brie Cheese	350	30
½ Bagel		

How to Order: "Bagel with Eggs and two orders Brie Cheese." Makes two meals.

1 Egg with Brie Cheese	350	24
Oatmeal Bar		

AU BON PAIN Women   Lunch/Dinner

Meal	Calories	Net Carbs
½ Turkey and Brie on a Plain Bagel	300	32
½ Chicken Breast Sandwich with Sundried Tomato Spread and Swiss Cheese on a Croissant	300	24
½ Tuna Sandwich with Cheddar Cheese on a Croissant	295	23
½ Chicken Caesar Wrap with Brie Cheese	375	29
½ Cobb Turkey Wrap with Swiss Cheese	365	30
½ Roast Beef Sandwich with Cheddar Cheese and Sundried Tomato Spread on Tomato Herb Bread	335	30

BAJA FRESH   Women   Lunch/Dinner

Tips:
+ Hold the chips.

Condiments:
+ Salsa: Have any kind, up to the maximum specified in the meal.
+ Cilantro: unlimited
+ Chilis: up to 1
+ Lemon slices: up to 2

MEAL	CALORIES	NET CARBS
Baja Fish Taco **Steak Taco**	334	21
Order with one tortilla per taco (2 tortillas total) With up to 3 containers of salsa	373	27
Chicken Taco Chilito (no sour cream)	331	29
Maximum salsa: 2 containers		
Steak Taco Chilito (no sour cream)	365	30
Maximum salsa: 2 containers		

Meal	Calories	Net Carbs
Baja Fish Taco	317	22
Chicken Taco 1 container salsa		
Order with one tortilla per taco (2 tortillas total) With up to 4 containers of salsa	356	31
½ Baja Chicken Burrito (no cheese, no chips)	350	30
With 1 container salsa	363	32
2 Shrimp Tacos	302	28
Order with just 3 tortillas With up to 2 containers of salsa	328	33
½ Chicken Taquitos with Beans (no sour cream)	360	23
With 1 container salsa	373	25
½ Chicken Enchiladas Verdes	380	36

Meal	Calories	Net Carbs
½ Chicken Enchiladas with Red Sauce (no sour cream)	385	36
½ Mini Steak Quesadita	350	33
Charbroiled Fish Taco Shrimp Taco Order with just 3 tortillas	372	34
Charbroiled Fish Taco Shrimp Taco 2 containers salsa Order with 1 tortilla per taco (2 tortillas total)	320	24
Charbroiled Fish Taco Chicken Taco 2 containers salsa Order with 1 tortilla per taco (2 tortillas total)	320	23

MEAL	CALORIES	NET CARBS
Baja Fish Taco	305	21
Shrimp Taco		
Order with one tortilla per taco (2 tortillas total)		
With up to 3 containers of salsa	344	28
Chicken Taco	302	30
Shrimp Taco		
Order with just 3 tortillas		
With 1 container of salsa	315	33

BLIMPIE Women   Lunch/Dinner

Tips for subs:
- ✦ Bread: white or wheat
- ✦ Cheese: any kind, unless specified otherwise
- ✦ Vegetables: any

MEAL	CALORIES	NET CARBS
¾ Steak & Onion Melt	330	35

MEAL	CALORIES	NET CARBS
¾ Golden Gate Gourmet Sandwich	300	29
Turkey Sub with Cheese (no mayo, no oil, discard ½ the bread)	305	25
Ham Sub with Cheese (no mayo, no oil, discard ½ the bread)	317	28
Tuna Sub with Cheese (no mayo, no oil, discard ½ the bread)	374	27
Club Sub with Cheese (no mayo, no oil, discard ½ the bread)	321	27

BOSTON MARKET   Women   Lunch/Dinner

Condiments:
+ Salt, pepper, Tabasco sauce: unlimited
+ Lemon wedges: up to 2
+ Ketchup: up to ½ soup spoon

MEAL	CALORIES	NET CARBS
⅓ One-Fourth White Chicken (with skin)	310	31
½ Cornbread (no butter) 1 side Fruit		

How to Order: "¼ White Chicken with 2
sides Fruit." (Comes with Cornbread.) Makes
two meals.

½ Turkey Breast	345	32

Green Beans
Stuffing

How to order: "Turkey Breast with Green
Beans and Stuffing, no Cornbread."

Snacks: Extra Turkey = 3 Proteins

½ Turkey Breast	325	30

2 soup spoons of Gravy
1 side Steamed Vegetables
½ Chocolate Chip Cookie

How to Order: "Turkey Breast with 2 sides
Steamed Vegetables, no Cornbread.
Chocolate Chip Cookie." Also ask for a soup
spoon. Makes two meals.

½ Turkey Breast	325	29

2 soup spoons of Gravy
1 side Steamed Vegetables
½ Oatmeal Scotchie Cookie

How to Order: "Turkey Breast with 2 sides
Steamed Vegetables, no Cornbread.

Oatmeal Scotchie Cookie." Also ask for a
soup spoon. Makes two meals.

| ½ Meatloaf | 285 | 20 |

Chicken Noodle Soup
Steamed Vegetables

How to Order: "Meatloaf with Chicken
Noodle Soup and Steamed Vegetables, no
Cornbread."

Snacks: Extra Meatloaf = 2 Proteins

| ½ Chicken Carver Sandwich | 320 | 29 |
| (with Cheese and Spread) | | |

| ½ Turkey Carver Sandwich | 315 | 30 |
| (with Cheese and Spread) | | |

| ½ Oriental Grilled Chicken Salad | 285 | 24 |
| (with dressing and noodles) | | |

| ½ of One-fourth White Chicken | 350 | 28 |
| (with skin) | | |

Vegetable Rice Pilaf
Green Beans

How to Order: "One-Fourth White Chicken
with Rice Pilaf and Green Beans, no
Cornbread."

Snacks: Extra chicken with skin = 3 Proteins

½ One-Fourth Dark Chicken   320   25
(with skin)

Cornbread (discard ½, no butter)
2 sides Steamed Vegetables

How to Order: "One-Fourth Dark Chicken
with 2 sides Steamed Vegetables." (Comes
with Cornbread.) Makes two meals.

Snacks: Extra chicken with skin = 3 Proteins

**½ of One-Fourth Dark
Chicken**   290   21
(remove skin)

½ Cornbread (no butter)
1 side Steamed Vegetables

How to Order: "One-Fourth Dark Chicken
with 2 sides Steamed Vegetables." (Comes
with Cornbread.)

BURGER KING Women   Breakfast

Tip: If milk size is 10 oz., drink ¾ of the amount listed
in the meal.

MEAL	CALORIES	NET CARBS
Croissant with Ham and Cheese (no Egg, discard ¼ the bread)	318	29
Milk (8 oz. low-fat) With 1 packet ketchup	328	32
Croissant with Ham and Cheese (no Egg)	360	35
Milk (8 oz. low-fat)		
Croissant with Ham & Egg (extra ham, no cheese)	345	24
With 1 packet ketchup	355	27
Egg Patty	300	26
2 containers Milk (8 oz. low-fat) With 1 packet ketchup	310	29

Meal	Calories	Net Carbs
Sourdough Breakfast Sandwich with Ham, Egg, and Cheese	380	28
¾ Croissant with Ham, Egg, and Cheese (extra ham, extra cheese)	338	21
1 packet ketchup		

BURGER KING Women Lunch/Dinner

Meal	Calories	Net Carbs
BK Veggie Burger (no mayo, no bun)	345	30
BK Veggie Burger with Cheese (no mayo, no bun)		
¼ Whopper with Cheese and Bacon (no mayo)	340	25
Cheeseburger	350	30
Whopper Jr. with Cheese (no mayo)	350	30

Meal	Calories	Net Carbs
Bacon Cheeseburger (discard ¼ the bun)	350	23

Meal	Calories	Net Carbs
½ Chicken Whopper with mayo	323	27

Side Salad
½ packet Fat-Free Ranch Dressing

Snacks: Extra ½ sandwich = 3 Snacks
extra chicken with mayo
(no bun) = 2 Proteins

Meal	Calories	Net Carbs
½ Chicken Whopper (no mayo)	280	30

Side Salad
½ Tomato Balsamic Vinaigrette Dressing
With ½ packet

	Calories	Net Carbs
Ranch Dressing	285	29

Snacks: Extra chicken = 2 Proteins

Meal	Calories	Net Carbs
Chicken Caesar Salad (no Parmesan cheese)	310	24

Sweet Onion Vinaigrette Dressing
With Tomato Balsamic

Vinaigrette Dressing	320	24
With Garden Ranch Dressing	330	23

8 Chicken Tenders	**358**	**24**
½ packet BBQ Sauce With ½ packet Sweet-and-Sour Sauce	360	25
With 1 BBQ Sauce	375	29
With 1 packet ketchup (instead of sauce)	350	23

¾ Double Hamburger (no cheese)	**330**	**22**

Original Chicken Sandwich (no mayo, discard ½ the bun)	**355**	**31**

Shrimp Caesar Salad	**290**	**23**
Parmesan Cheese Toast (comes with salad) Fat-Free Ranch Dressing		
With Sweet Onion Vinaigrette Dressing	350	24
With Tomato Balsamic Vinaigrette Dressing	360	24
With Garden Ranch Dressing	370	23

CARL'S JR.   Women   Breakfast

MEAL	CALORIES	NET CARBS
Side of Scrambled Eggs	375	26
Side of Bacon		
¾ of 10 oz. Orange Juice		
¾ Sourdough Breakfast Sandwich with Ham	338	29
Sourdough Breakfast Sandwich (no meat, discard ¼ the bread)	362	29
¾ Sourdough Breakfast Sandwich with Bacon	353	28
Side of Scrambled Eggs	373	27
Side of *Swiss* Cheese (on the Eggs)		
English Muffin (no margarine)		
Side of Scrambled Eggs	363	24
Side of Bacon		
⅔ of 10 oz. Orange Juice		
With 1 packet ketchup	373	27

MEAL	CALORIES	NET CARBS
Side of Scrambled Eggs	368	27
Side of Bacon		
English Muffin (no margarine)		

CARL'S JR.   Women   Lunch/Dinner

MEAL	CALORIES	NET CARBS
½ Charbroiled Santa Fe Chicken Sandwich (with everything)	305	21
½ Chili Burger	345	26
6-piece Chicken Stars	345	24
½ Milk (10 oz.)		
With ½ packet BBQ Sauce	370	30
With ½ packet Mustard Sauce	370	30
With ½ packet Sweet-and-Sour Sauce	370	30
Famous Star Hamburger (no mayo, remove ½ the bread)	343	28

MEAL	CALORIES	NET CARBS
½ Charbroiled Chicken Salad-to-Go	320	25
⅓ Onion Rings ½ packet Fat-Free Italian Dressing		
Instructions: Each person eats ⅓ onion rings. Discard any remaining onion rings before beginning meal. Split the salad and dressing packet.		
With 1 packet ketchup per person	330	28
½ Charbroiled Chicken Salad-to-Go	333	23
½ Fried Zucchini ½ packet Fat-Free Italian Dressing With 1 packet ketchup per person	343	26
Famous Star Hamburger (no mayo, no ketchup, remove ½ the bread)	324	24
½ Charbroiled Chicken Salad-to-Go	310	23
½ Small Fries With ½ packet Fat-Free		

Italian Dressing	318	25
With 1 packet ketchup		
per person	320	26

CHICK-FIL-A Women   Lunch/Dinner

MEAL	CALORIES	NET CARBS
Chargrilled Chicken		
Garden Salad	305	30
(don't eat the sunflower seeds—save for a snack)		
Croutons		
Fat-Free Honey Mustard Dijon Dressing		
With Reduced-Fat Raspberry		
Vinaigrette Dressing	330	31
Chargrilled Chicken		
Garden Salad	355	29
(don't eat the sunflower seeds—save for a snack)		
½ packet Light Italian Dressing		
½ Brownie		
Chick-fil-A Chicken Salad		
Sandwich on Wheat Bread	350	28

MEAL	CALORIES	NET CARBS
½ Chick-n-Strips	355	28

½ Small Waffle Potato Fries
1 Side Salad
½ packet Light Italian Dressing

Each person orders their own side salad.
Split Chick-n-Strips, Waffle Potato Fries, and
dressing

With 1 packet ketchup	365	31
¾ Chicken Deluxe Sandwich	315	28
¾ Chick-fil-A Chicken Sandwich	285	27

CHILI'S   Women   Lunch/Dinner*

MEAL	CALORIES	NET CARBS
1 Cup Chicken Enchilada Soup	293	20

Dinner Caesar Salad (no dressing)

*Net carbohydrates were calculated using estimated dietary fiber
based on similar ingredients, since dietary fiber information was
not available at the time of this writing.

Vinegar or lemon wedges for dressing
(on the side)

Option 1: Order as Soup and Salad Combo.
Ask that the soup come in a cup rather than
a bowl.

Option 2: Order as Soup and Salad Combo.
The soup will come in a bowl (twice as
much as a cup). Eat half the soup with the
salad. Take the other half home. Make a
second meal from extra soup and your own
salad.

With 1 soup spoon of Low-Fat Vinaigrette Dressing (ordered on the side)	312	28

½ Lettuce Wraps (use the sauces that come with it)	365	26

½ Grilled Baby Back Ribs with ½ Cinnamon Apples (no Fries)	333	21
With Vegetables (no butter) no Fries (Eat ½ Vegetables)	352	29

MEAL	CALORIES	NET CARBS
½ Guiltless Grill Chicken Pita	313	31
1 tsp. Olive Oil (add to the pita)		
½ Guiltless Grill Chicken Sandwich	304	28
1 tsp. Olive Oil (add to the sandwich)		
½ Half-Turkey Sandwich (no Fries)	321	21
½ Chicken Enchilada Soup ½ Vegetables (no butter)		

How to Order: "Turkey Combo with Chicken Enchilada Soup, and Vegetables (no butter) instead of fries." Makes two meals.

½ Oldtimer Burger (no Fries, no butter on bun, discard ¼ the bun)	347	21
2 tsp. ketchup (per person)		
With Vegetables (no butter) instead of Fries (split the Vegetables)	367	26
Bowl Chicken Tortilla Soup	274	23

Meal	Calories	Net Carbs
Cup Chicken Tortilla Soup	346	31
Beans		
Vegetables		
¼ **Chicken Fajita Quesadilla**	305	20
⅓ **Ginger-Citrus Glazed Salmon**	326	27
1 order Garlic Toast		

How to Order: "Ginger-Citrus Glazed
Salmon with 2 orders Garlic Toast instead of
side dishes." Makes two meals.

Snacks: Extra ⅓ salmon = 2 Proteins

Bowl Tortilla Soup	290	25

Caesar Salad (no croutons, no dressing)
Vinegar or lemon wedges for dressing

How to Order: "Soup and Salad Combo with
Tortilla Soup and Caesar Salad (no croutons,
no dressing), vinegar or lemon wedges."

½ **Grilled Chicken Caribbean Salad**	325	31
½ **Grilled Chicken Caesar Salad**	330	23

CHURCH'S CHICKEN   Women Lunch/Dinner

Tips:
+ No biscuits or butter with meals

Condiments:
+ Jalapeños: up to 1

MEAL	CALORIES	NET CARBS
Wing	340	21
Mashed Potatoes with Gravy		
2 Krispy Tender Strips	303	27
1 packet BBQ Sauce		
Breast	368	26
1 packet BBQ Sauce Corn on the Cob		
With 1 packet Sweet-and-Sour Sauce (instead of BBQ Sauce)	370	27
Breast	319	24
1 packet BBQ Sauce Mashed Potatoes with Gravy		
With 1 packet Sweet-and-Sour Sauce (instead of BBQ Sauce)	321	25

MEAL	CALORIES	NET CARBS
Thigh	369	20
Corn on the Cob		
Leg	371	23
Coleslaw		
Corn on the Cob		

DAIRY QUEEN Women   Lunch/Dinner

MEAL	CALORIES	NET CARBS
Cheeseburger	340	27
½ Double Cheeseburger	375	25
½ Chocolate Dilly Bar		
½ Grilled Chicken Salad	375	25
¼ packet Fat-Free Ranch Dressing		
Hot Dog		
Grilled Chicken Sandwich	340	24
With 1 packet ketchup	350	27
Crispy Chicken Salad	375	21
1 packet Fat-Free Ranch Dressing		

DEL TACO Women

Lunch/Dinner

Tips:
+ If milk is 10 oz., drink ¾ of the amount specified in the meal.

MEAL	CALORIES	NET CARBS
½ Del Beef Burrito ½ Chicken Taco Del Carbon	360	28
½ Del Beef Burrito ½ Milk (8 oz. low-fat)	340	27
Chicken Taco Del Carbon Carnitas Taco	350	33
Chicken Taco Del Carbon Soft Taco	330	32
Chicken Soft Taco Soft Taco	370	30
Chicken Taco Del Carbon Taco	330	27

MEAL	CALORIES	NET CARBS
¾ Carnitas Burrito	330	29
Snacks: Extra ¼ burrito = 1 Snack		
Chicken Soft Taco	340	30
Milk (8 oz.)		
Steak Taco Del Carbon	350	32
Milk (8 oz. low-fat)		
Chicken Taco Del Carbon	300	32
Milk (8 oz.)		
Carnitas Taco	300	31
Milk (8 oz. low-fat)		
Ultimate Taco	358	22
¾ of 8-oz. Milk		

DENNY'S Women   Breakfast

Tips:

+ Syrup: use regular, *not* sugar-free
+ Eggs: order any style
+ Try Tabasco sauce on eggs

Condiments:

+ Salt, pepper, Tabasco sauce, mustard, and
  vinegar: unlimited
+ Ketchup: up to 1 teaspoon
+ Half-and-half: up to ½ container

MEAL	CALORIES	NET CARBS
1 Egg (easy on the oil)	364	32
Cheese (on or in the egg) Oatmeal (no sugar, no butter) With 3 tsp. milk	374	33
2 Eggs with Cheese (easy on the oil)	357	25

Fruit Salad
½ English Muffin (no butter, no jelly)

How to Order: "Original Grand Slam. On the
eggs, go easy on the oil. Cheese on or in the
eggs, no meat, Fruit instead of pancakes,
English Muffin, no butter."

2 Eggbeaters	311	29
1 piece Bacon 1 piece Sausage 1 Pancake (no butter) 3 tsp. syrup		

How to Order: "Original Grand Slam with Eggbeaters, just 1 piece of Bacon and 1 piece of Sausage, 1 Pancake, no butter."

2 Eggs (easy on the oil)　　　366　　　29

2 pieces Bacon
1 Pancake (no butter)
3 tsp. syrup

How to Order: "Original Grand Slam. On the eggs, go easy on the oil. No sausage, just 1 pancake, no butter."

2 Eggbeaters with Cheese　292　　　31
(on or in the Eggbeaters)

1 Pancake (no butter)
3 tsp. syrup

How to Order: "Original Grand Slam with Eggbeaters. Cheese on or in the Eggbeaters, no meat, just 1 pancake, no butter."

2 Eggbeaters with Cheese　335　　　31
(on or in the Eggbeaters)

1 piece Bacon
1 Pancake (no butter)
3 tsp. syrup

How to Order: "Original Grand Slam with Eggbeaters. Cheese on or in the Eggbeaters.

No sausage, just 1 piece of Bacon, 1 Pancake, no butter."

2 Eggbeaters with Cheese (on or in the Eggbeaters)	335	25

1 Biscuit (no butter)

How to Order: "Original Grand Slam with Eggbeaters. Cheese on or in the Eggbeaters, no Hash Browns, 1 Biscuit, no butter."

2 Eggbeaters	275	31

2 pieces Bacon
English Muffin (no butter)
½ package Jelly

How to Order: "Original Grand Slam with Eggbeaters, no sausage. Instead of pancakes, an English Muffin, no butter."

2 Eggbeaters	360	24

1 piece Bacon
1 piece Sausage
English Muffin (no butter, no jelly)

How to Order: "Original Grand Slam with Eggbeaters, just 1 piece of Bacon, 1 piece of Sausage. Instead of pancakes, an English Muffin, no butter."

MEAL	CALORIES	NET CARBS
2 Eggs (easy on the oil)	331	25

½ Bagel
½ package Cream Cheese

How to Order: "Original Grand Slam. On the
Eggs, go easy on the oil. No meat. Instead of
Pancakes, a Bagel with Cream Cheese."

2 Eggbeaters	333	24

2 pieces Bacon
1 Biscuit (no butter)

How to Order: "Original Grand Slam with
Eggbeaters, no Sausage. Instead of
Pancakes, just 1 Biscuit, no butter."

With ½ package jelly on the biscuit	352	29

2 Eggbeaters	338	21

2 pieces Bacon
Hash Browns

How to Order: "Original Grand Slam with
Eggbeaters, no sausage. Instead of
pancakes, Hash Browns."

MEAL	CALORIES	NET CARBS
2 Eggs with Cheese (easy on the oil)	368	29

1 Pancake (no butter)
3 tsp. syrup

How to Order: "Original Grand Slam. On the eggs, go easy on the oil. Cheese on or in the eggs, no meat, just 1 Pancake, no butter."

2 Eggbeaters with Cheese (on or in the Eggbeaters)	306	27

½ Bagel
½ package Cream Cheese

How to Order: "Original Grand Slam with Eggbeaters. Cheese on or in the Eggbeaters, no meat. Instead of Pancakes, a Bagel with Cream Cheese."

2 Eggbeaters	304	30

3 pieces Bacon
1 Pancake (no butter)
3 tsp. syrup

How to Order: "Original Grand Slam with Eggbeaters. Instead of sausage, 3 pieces of Bacon, and just one Pancake, no butter."

MEAL	CALORIES	NET CARBS
1 Egg (easy on the oil)	287	31

½ piece Ham
1 piece Bacon
1 Pancake (no butter)
3 tsp. syrup

How to Order: "Original Grand Slam. On the Eggs, go easy on the oil. Ham instead of Sausage, and just 2 Pancakes (no butter)." Makes two meals.

1 Egg (easy on the oil)	281	27

½ piece Ham
1 piece Bacon
½ Bagel (no butter)

How to Order: "Original Grand Slam. On the Eggs, go easy on the oil. Ham instead of Sausage, and a Bagel instead of Pancakes." Makes two meals.

With ½ packet Cream Cheese	331	28
With ½ packet jelly	299	32

MEAL	CALORIES	NET CARBS
1 Egg (easy on the oil)	326	25

½ piece Ham
1 piece Bacon
½ Hash Browns
½ English Muffin

How to Order: "Original Grand Slam. On the
Eggs, go easy on the oil. Ham instead of
Sausage, Hash Browns instead of Pancakes,
and an English Muffin, no butter." Makes
two meals.

With ½ package jelly	343	30
1 Eggbeater with Cheese (on or in the Eggbeater)	361	30

1 piece Bacon
1 piece Sausage
1 Pancake (no butter)
3 tsp. syrup

How to Order: "Original Grand Slam with
Eggbeaters, double Cheese on or in the
Eggbeaters, just 2 Pancakes, no butter."
Makes 2 meals.

MEAL	CALORIES	NET CARBS
1 Eggbeater with Cheese (on or in the Eggbeater)	356	26

1 piece Bacon
1 piece Sausage
½ Bagel (no butter, no Cream Cheese)

How to Order: "Original Grand Slam with Eggbeaters, double Cheese on or in the Eggbeaters, a Bagel instead of Pancakes, no butter." Makes two meals.

With ½ teaspoon jelly	363	31

2 Eggs (easy on the oil)	313	24

¾ bowl Oatmeal (no sugar, no butter)

How to Order: "2 Eggs, easy on the oil with Oatmeal, no butter."

With 3 tsp. milk	321	25

Tip: Discard the sugar that comes with the Oatmeal. Fill the empty sugar container with Oatmeal and set it aside (but don't eat it). What's left in the bowl is ¾ of the Oatmeal.

MEAL	CALORIES	NET CARBS
1 Egg with Cheese (easy on the oil)	368	29

2 pieces Bacon
1 Pancake (no butter)
3 tsp. syrup

How to Order: "Original Grand Slam with just
one Egg, easy on the oil, with Cheese, no
Sausage, just 1 Pancake, no butter"

DENNY'S Women   Lunch

Tips:
+ Vegetable Beef Soup is currently offered on
  Saturday, Sunday, and Monday.

MEAL	CALORIES	NET CARBS
1 Chicken Strip	352	26

2 Mozzarella Sticks
½ container marinara sauce
½ serving Tomato Slices

How to Order: "The Sampler, with Tomatoes
instead of Onion Rings, and no Ranch
Sauce." Makes two meals.

MEAL	CALORIES	NET CARBS

**½ Grilled Chicken Breast
Salad**   321   22

1 piece Garlic Toast (comes with salad)

Instructions: To make this into 2 meals,
order an extra piece of Garlic Toast. Eat as
many vegetables as you like, but eat ½ of
the cheese and ½ of the chicken. Eat the
salad dry, with vinegar, or with one of these
dressings:

With Low-Calorie Italian Dressing	336	25
With Fat-Free Ranch Dressing	346	28

½ Turkey Breast Salad   373   29
(no cheese, no bread, no dressing)

½ piece of Cheesecake (plain)

Instructions: Eat the salad dry, with vinegar,
or with lemon wedges. (This meal contains
17.5 g protein, 1 g less than the cutoff but
still enough to be filling.)

½ Albacore Tuna Melt   356   21

½ dish Cottage Cheese (instead of Fries)

MEAL	CALORIES	NET CARBS
½ Classic Burger (no toasting oil)	281	26
No Fries (can substitute Tomatoes)		
With Tomatoes	294	28

Snacks: Extra meat without bread = 2 Proteins (with fat)

½ Ham & Swiss Sandwich on Rye (no mayo)	352	35

½ Side Salad (no croutons)
¾ Small Milk

How to Order: "Sandwich and Salad Combo, with Ham & Swiss Sandwich, no mayo, no croutons on the salad, vinegar (or Low-Calorie Italian Dressing) on the side, small milk." Makes two meals.

Instructions: Eat the salad dry, with vinegar, or with 3 teaspoons Low-Calorie Italian Dressing. To make this into 2 meals, order 2 small milks.

With 3 teaspoons Low-Calorie Italian Dressing	359	36

½ Ham & Swiss Sandwich on Rye (no mayo)	288	26

Vegetable Beef Soup

How to Order: "Sandwich and Soup Combo.
Ham and Swiss Sandwich, no mayo,
Vegetable Beef Soup."

Instructions: To make this into 2 meals,
order an extra bowl of soup.

½ Boca Burger (no toasting oil)	270	29

½ Cottage Cheese (instead of Fries)

½ Boca Burger (no toasting oil)	293	29

1 double order Cheese (on Burger)
No Fries (can substitute Tomato slices)

With American Cheese	293	29
With Swiss Cheese	302	29
With Cheddar Cheese	324	28
With Tomatoes instead of Fries	315	32

¾ Super Bird Sandwich (no mayo, no toasting oil)	373	25

No Fries (can substitute Tomato Slices)

Snacks: Extra ¼ sandwich = 1 Snack

MEAL	CALORIES	NET CARBS
¾ Grilled Chicken Breast Salad (no cheese)	**279**	**25**

½ piece Garlic Toast (comes with salad)
Fruit Salad

Instructions: Eat as many vegetables as you like, but eat ¾ of the chicken. Eat the salad dry, with vinegar, or with one of these dressings (ordered on the side):

With ½ container Low-Calorie Italian Dressing	294	31
With ½ container Fat-Free Ranch Dressing	304	33

½ Ham & Swiss on Rye	**300**	**25**

½ Cottage Cheese (instead of Fries)
½ Side Salad

With 3 tsp. Low-Calorie Italian Dressing	308	26
With 3 tsp. Fat-Free Ranch Dressing	313	28
With 3 tsp. French Dressing	353	27

½ Super Bird Sandwich	**361**	**28**

Cottage Cheese (instead of Fries)
Fruit Salad

Instructions: To make this into 2 meals,
order an extra bowl of cottage cheese and
an extra fruit salad.

½ Club Sandwich   318   22
(no mayo)

Double order Swiss Cheese (on sandwich)

No Fries (can substitute Tomatoes)

With American Cheese   309   22
With Cheddar Cheese   340   21
With Tomatoes   331   24

**Turkey Breast Sandwich on
whole wheat**   321   34
(no mayo, discard ¼ the bread)

Salad (no croutons)
3 tsp. Ranch Dressing

How to order: "Sandwich and Salad Combo,
with Turkey Sandwich, no mayo. Salad with
Ranch (or Caesar or Blue Cheese) Dressing
on the side."

With 3 tsp. Caesar Dressing   323   34
With 3 tsp. Blue Cheese   342   32

Chicken Strip Salad   322   23
(no cheese, eat ½ the chicken pieces)

Fat-Free Ranch Dressing

½ Garlic Toast (comes with salad)

Snacks: Extra chicken pieces = 2 Snacks

DENNY'S   Women   Dinner

Tips:

+ Vegetable Beef Soup is currently offered on
  Saturday, Sunday, and Monday.
+ Senior meals are for guests age 55 and older.

MEAL	CALORIES	NET CARBS
½ Turkey with ½ Stuffing and ½ Gravy (no bread)	295	35
Side Salad 3 tsp. Ranch, Caesar, or Blue Cheese Dressing on the side		
Instructions: To make this into 2 meals, order the Turkey Dinner with 2 side salads. Each person gets her or his own salad. Otherwise, order 1 salad.		
With 3 tsp. Ranch Dressing	295	35
With 3 tsp. Caesar Dressing	297	35
With 3 tsp. Blue Cheese Dressing	322	35

*Snacks: Extra turkey (without stuffing or gravy) = 3
Proteins*

½ Turkey with ½ Stuffing and ½ Gravy (no bread)	301	34

½ Tomatoes
½ Side Salad
3 tsp. dressing on the side (one of the
following):

With 3 tsp. Ranch Dressing	301	34
With 3 tsp. Caesar Dressing	303	34
With 3 tsp. Blue Cheese Dressing	318	34

Seniors Only	304	31

Senior Fried Shrimp Dinner (no bread)
Cottage Cheese
Corn

With ½ container marinara sauce	328	35

Fried Shrimp Dinner (no bread, eat 7 shrimp)	330	31

Carrots
Green Beans
With 1 container marinara sauce

Snacks: Extra 3 shrimp (with or without marinara sauce) = 1 Snack

Seniors Only	**299**	**27**
Senior Fried Shrimp Dinner (no bread)		
Cottage Cheese		
Carrots		
With 1 container marinara sauce		

½ Fried Shrimp Dinner	**286**	**30**
(5 shrimp, no bread)		
With ½ container marinara sauce		
½ Cottage Cheese		
½ Mashed Potatoes		
½ Side Salad		
With 3 tsp. Ranch Dressing	318	30
With 3 tsp. Caesar Dressing	319	30
With 3 tsp. Blue Cheese		
Dressing	328	30

½ Pot Roast with ½ Gravy	**335**	**24**
(no bread)		
Carrots		
Fruit		
Side Salad (no croutons)		
3 tsp. dressing on the side (one of the following):		

With 3 tsp. Ranch Dressing	335	24
With 3 tsp. Caesar Dressing	337	24
With 3 tsp. Blue Cheese Dressing	352	24

Snacks: Extra pot roast (with or without gravy) = 3 Proteins

½ Pot Roast with Gravy (no bread)	301	26

½ Fruit
½ Seasoned Fries

Substitute Onion Rings instead of Seasoned Fries	361	27

Seniors Only	328	26

¾ Senior Pot Roast with ¾ Gravy
Mashed Potatoes
Green Beans

Snack: Extra Pot Roast (with or without gravy) = 1 Protein

Sirloin Steak Dinner	346	25

½ Steak and ½ Baked Potato (plain)
1 container Cottage Cheese

With a side salad (no croutons), eaten dry or with vinegar or lemon wedges	371	29

Tip: Try cottage cheese on the potato.

Snacks: Extra steak = 2 Proteins

Fish & Chips Dinner   353   26
(2 pieces fish, no Fries, no tartar sauce, no bread)

½ Cottage Cheese
Fruit Salad

Instructions: If splitting the meal, order a second bowl of fruit for the other person.

Tip: Try vinegar on the fish.

Snacks: 1 piece fish = 1 Snack

2 pieces Chicken Strip Dinner 342   33
(no sauce, no bread)

½ Fruit Bowl

Tip: Try vinegar or mustard on the chicken strips.

Einstein Bros. Bagels   Women   Breakfast

Tips:

+ Bagel sandwiches were calculated on plain bagels. You can substitute other bagels; if you do, calories and net carbohydrates will vary slightly. These meals are designed to be eaten with the regular bagels, not the low-carb bagels.

Meal	Calories	Net Carbs
Lox and Cream Cheese Sandwich (on Artisan Wheat Bread instead of a Bagel, order cream cheese on the side, use 1 soup spoon of cream cheese, discard ¼ the bread)	325	33
With 2 soup spoons of cream cheese	360	32
½ Santa Fe Egg Frittata (discard ¼ the bread)	320	30
½ Sausage and Egg Frittata (discard ¼ the bread)	290	28
½ Bacon and Egg Frittata (on Artisan Wheat Bread instead of a Bagel)	380	22
½ Denver Omelette Breakfast Panini	375	34

EINSTEIN BROS. BAGELS   Women Lunch/Dinner

Tip:

+ When a meal says "no chips," you may substitute a piece of fruit for the chips. However,
  don't eat the fruit with your meal. Save it for
  making snacks (see page 35).

Condiments:

+ Pickles: up to 1

MEAL	CALORIES	NET CARBS
½ Albacore Tuna Sandwich on Artisan Wheat Bread (discard ¼ the bread) 1 cup Clam Chowder (no Lahvash Bread)	360	33
½ Roast Turkey Sandwich on Artisan Wheat Bread (no chips)	305	23
½ Ham & Cheese Panini Sandwich (no chips)	320	33
Bowl Turkey Chili (no Lahvash Bread)	330	28

Meal	Calories	Net Carbs
½ Tasty Turkey Sandwich on Asiago Cheese Bagel (no chips, add cheddar or Swiss cheese, discard ¼ the bread)	310	32
½ Italian Chicken Panini Sandwich (no chips)	345	33
½ Black Forest Ham on Challah (no chips)	310	31
½ Black Forest Ham on Challah (discard ¼ the bread) ½ Bros. Bistro Salad (no nuts, no Lahvash Bread, use soup spoon of dressing on the side)	373	28
½ Tasty Turkey Sandwich on Asiago Cheese Bagel (discard ¼ the bread) ½ Bros. Bistro Salad (no nuts, no Lahvash Bread, use ½ soup spoon of dressing on the side)	370	35

MEAL	CALORIES	NET CARBS
½ Albacore Tuna Sandwich on Artisan Wheat Bread	300	26
½ Bros. Bistro Salad (no nuts, no Lahvash Bread, use ½ soup spoon of dressing on the side)		
½ Roasted Turkey Sandwich on Artisan Wheat Bread	340	26
½ Bros. Bistro Salad (no cheese, no nuts, no Lahvash Bread, use ½ soup spoon of dressing on the side)		
½ Black Forest Ham on Challah (extra cheese, no chips)	350	32
½ Chipotle Chicken Salad (no dressing)	355	25
½ Lahvash Bread (comes with the salad)		
How to Order: "Chipotle Chicken Salad, no dressing." Makes two meals.		
Cup Turkey Chili	335	28
½ Bros. Bistro Salad (no nuts, use ½ soup spoon of dressing on the side) ½ piece of Lahvash Bread (comes with the salad)		

El Pollo Loco   Women   Lunch/Dinner

Condiments:

+ Salsa: 1 to 2 containers at your discretion (see calories and net carbs below)
+ Jalapeños: up to 1
+ Jalapeño sauce packets: up to 1
+ Lemon wedges: up to 2

Salsa	Calories (in 1 container)	Net Carbs (in 1 container)
House	6	1
Spicy Chipotle	7	1
Pico de Gallo	10	1
Avocado	20	1

Meal	Calories	Net Carbs
Leg	355	21
1 container Fresh Vegetables		
Churro		
With 1 container		
Avocado Salsa	375	21
½ Flame-Grilled Chicken Breast	327	32
Fresh Vegetables		
Kid's Size Foster's Freeze Soft-Serve Ice Cream		

Meal	Calories	Net Carbs
½ Flame-Grilled Chicken Breast	346	21
Fresh Vegetables		
1 Churro		
Leg	336	32
Fresh Vegetables		
Kid's Size Foster's Freeze Soft-Serve Ice Cream		
Leg	276	21
Fresh Vegetables		
1 Corn Cobbette		
1 container Avocado Salsa		
With 1 Avocado Salsa +		
1 Pico de Gallo	296	23
½ Chicken Quesadilla	367	26
Fresh Vegetables		
½ Chicken Lover's Burrito	333	29
Fresh Vegetables		
With 1 container		
Pico de Gallo	353	31
With 1 container Avocado		
Salsa	373	31

MEAL	CALORIES	NET CARBS
Leg	372	27
Coleslaw		
1 Corn Cobbette		
Popcorn Chicken	307	32
1 Corn Cobbette		
½ Flame-Grilled Chicken Breast	358	29
½ Macaroni and Cheese		
1 Corn Cobbette		
Thigh	287	21
Mashed Potatoes (no gravy)		
Fresh Vegetables		
With 1 container Pico de Gallo	307	23
With 1 container Avocado Salsa	327	23

HARDEE'S Women   Breakfast

MEAL	CALORIES	NET CARBS
Ham, Egg, and Cheese Biscuit (discard ½ the Biscuit)	375	21

MEAL	CALORIES	NET CARBS
¾ Sunrise Croissant with Ham (add extra Swiss Cheese)	360	21
Tortilla Scrambler (add Swiss Cheese and 1 packet ketchup)	370	21
¾ Sunrise Croissant with Ham (add extra American Cheese)	360	22
Croissant Sandwich with Ham and Cheese (no American Cheese, keep Swiss Cheese, discard ¼ bread)	331	21
Croissant and Ham Sandwich (no cheese, extra Ham)	376	28
Chicken Fillet Biscuit (no biscuit) Grits	340	31
Frisco Breakfast Sandwich	360	36
Croissant Sandwich with Ham and Cheese	354	27

(ask for both pieces to be Swiss Cheese
rather than American Cheese, no egg)

¾ Sunrise Croissant with Ham (add Bacon)	368	21
With 1 packet ketchup on sandwich	375	23

Croissant Sandwich with Ham and Cheese   346   28
(no American Cheese, no Egg, keep the
Swiss Cheese, extra Ham)

HARDEE'S Women   Lunch/Dinner

MEAL	CALORIES	NET CARBS
Regular Roast Beef Sandwich	304	27
If made with butter	334	27
1½ Slammers	360	29

Snacks: Extra ½ Slammer = 1 Snack

½ Grilled Sourdough Burger with Bacon and Onions (no mayo, no cheese)	372	21

MEAL	CALORIES	NET CARBS
½ Grilled Sourdough Burger with Swiss Cheese and Onions (no mayo, no bacon, no American Cheese)	374	21
½ Charbroiled Chicken Sandwich with Mayo (Add Swiss Cheese)	320	25
½ Big Chicken Sandwich (no mayo, no butter, add Swiss Cheese)	315	37
Slammer with Cheese (add Swiss Cheese) Sandwich will contain 1 piece Swiss Cheese and 1 piece American Cheese	330	20
Slammer with 2 Pieces Swiss Cheese 1 packet ketchup	350	21
½ Big Hot Ham 'n Cheese Sandwich (extra Swiss Cheese)	310	28
Fried Chicken Leg with Gravy ⅔ Milk 10 oz.	290	30

MEAL	CALORIES	NET CARBS
½ Low-Carb Charbroiled Grilled Chicken Club (no gravy)	300	22
Small Mashed Potatoes		

IN-N-OUT Women   Lunch/Dinner

Condiments:
+ Onions on burgers (raw)

MEAL	CALORIES	NET CARBS
¾ Double Meat Burger (mustard & ketchup instead of Spread)	300	31
Snacks: Extra ¼ sandwich = 1 Snack		
¾ Double Meat Burger	375	29
Snacks: Extra ¼ sandwich = 1 Snack		
Protein-Style Double Meat Burger (mustard and ketchup instead of Spread, remove ½ of one meat patty)	333	23
⅓ container Fries		

With 2 tsp. ketchup	343	26
With 4 tsp. ketchup	353	29

Snacks: Extra meat = 1 Protein

Cheeseburger	**362**	**31**

(mustard and ketchup instead of spread,
discard ¼ the bread)

JACK IN THE BOX　Women　Lunch/Dinner

MEAL	CALORIES	NET CARBS
Cheeseburger	**360**	**30**
½ Zesty Turkey Pannido Sandwich	**370**	**25**
Chicken Club Salad	**335**	

(no almonds—save them for a snack)

½ packet Low-Fat Balsamic Vinaigrette Dressing
Croutons

Discard ½ the Cheese
Discard ½ the Bacon

¾ Hamburger with extra meat	**345**	**22**

Snacks: Extra ¼ hamburger = 1 Snack

MEAL	CALORIES	NET CARBS
Asian Chicken Salad	335	27

Wonton Strips
½ Almonds (discard extras before
beginning meal)
½ packet Low-Fat Balsamic Vinaigrette Dressing

Asian Chicken Salad	345	22

½ Wonton Strips (discard extras before
beginning meal)
Almonds
½ packet Low-Fat Balsamic Vinaigrette Dressing

Southwest Chicken Salad	300	22

(no Spicy Corn Sticks, remove ½ the Chicken)

½ packet Low-Fat Balsamic Vinaigrette Dressing

With ½ Corn Sticks (discard extras		
before beginning meal)	365	32

With ⅓ packet Southwest Dressing
(no Corn Sticks, no Low-Fat Balsamic

Vinaigrette Dressing)	370	22

Snacks: Extra Chicken = 1 Protein

Chicken Fajita Pita	330	32
With marinara sauce	345	35

MEAL	CALORIES	NET CARBS
½ Roasted Turkey Sandwich	315	25
½ Side Salad (no croutons)		
With ½ packet Low-Fat Balsamic Vinaigrette Dressing	335	28
½ Philly Cheesesteak Sandwich	335	30
½ Side Salad (no croutons) ½ Low-Fat Vinaigrette Dressing		
Breakfast Jack with *Triple Ham*	350	32
½ Ultimate Club Sandwich (no sauce)	290	24
With sauce	320	24

KFC Women   Lunch/Dinner

Tips:

✦ Hold the biscuit unless it's listed with the meal below.

✦ Chicken and sides can be ordered à la carte.

MEAL	CALORIES	NET CARBS
Drumstick (Extra Crispy)	360	29
Macaroni and Cheese		
Small Corn (or ½ Large Corn)		
Drumstick (Original Recipe)	340	28
Macaroni and Cheese		
Small Corn (or ½ Large Corn)		
4 Honey BBQ Sauced Wings	343	28
(you can order the 6-piece and save 2 for snacks)		
Snacks: Each extra wing = 1 Snack		
½ Tender Crisp Sandwich	335	21
(with sauce)		
Honey BBQ Sandwich	268	30
(discard ¼ the bread—take it from the bottom)		
Tender Roast Sandwich	344	23
(remove ¼ the chicken)		
Snacks: Extra chicken = 1 Protein		
Drumstick (Original Recipe)	333	24
Green Beans		
¾ Biscuit (no butter)		

MEAL	CALORIES	NET CARBS
Drumstick (Extra Crispy) Macaroni and Cheese Green Beans	340	22
½ Twister Wrap (made with Roasted Chicken Strip) 1 order Green Beans How to Order: "A Twister Wrap made with a Roasted Chicken Strip, 2 sides of Green Beans." Makes two meals.	325	28
Popcorn Chicken (Kid's Size) 2 orders Green Beans	370	22
Wing (Extra Crispy) 2 orders Green Beans ½ Biscuit (no butter)	370	28
Drumstick (Extra Crispy) 2 orders Green Beans ½ Biscuit (no butter)	340	23
½ Tender Roast Sandwich (with sauce) ½ order Baked Beans	310	31

LONG JOHN SILVER'S Women Lunch/Dinner

Tips:

+ When ordering fish or chicken, ask for "no Fried Crumbs." Discard any that come with the meal.
+ Fish pieces are shaped like diamonds. Chicken pieces are smaller, with an irregular shape.

Condiments:

+ Ketchup: up to 1 packet (unless the meal says otherwise)
+ Cocktail sauce: up to 1 packet (unless the meal says otherwise)
+ Vinegar: unlimited

MEAL	CALORIES	NET CARBS
1 Fish Piece	370	25
1 Chicken Piece		
Don't add ketchup or cocktail sauce.		
2 Chicken Pieces	370	29
Corn Cobbette		
Don't add ketchup or cocktail sauce.		

MEAL	CALORIES	NET CARBS
Shrimp & Seafood Salad (no dressing)	330	26
With ½ packet Lite Italian Dressing	340	28
Don't add ketchup or cocktail sauce.		

Shrimp & Seafood Salad (no croutons, no Fried Crumbs, no dressing)	300	28

2 Hushpuppies

Tip: Use malt vinegar for dressing.

Don't add ketchup or cocktail sauce.

Shrimp & Seafood Salad (no croutons, no Fried Crumbs, no dressing)	340	22
2 pieces Giant Shrimp		
With ½ packet Lite Italian Dressing	350	24
With 1 packet cocktail sauce (or ketchup)	357	26

Shrimp & Seafood Salad (no croutons, no Fried Crumbs, no dressing)	320	23

3 Cheesesticks

With ½ packet		
Lite Italian Dressing	330	25
With ½ packet		
Fat-Free French Dressing	345	29

McDONALD'S Women   Breakfast

MEAL	CALORIES	NET CARBS
Scrambled Eggs	365	22
2 pieces Canadian Bacon		
Hash Browns		
Apple Dippers (no dipping sauce)		
With 1 packet ketchup	375	25
Scrambled Eggs	310	26
Canadian Bacon		
Snack-size Fruit and Yogurt Parfait (discard Granola)		
With 1 packet ketchup	320	29
With Granola on Parfait	340	31
Bacon, Egg & Cheese Biscuit	350	23
(no bacon, discard ¼ the bread)		

2 pieces Canadian Bacon
With 1 packet ketchup   360   26

Bacon, Egg & Cheese Biscuit   360   23
(no Cheese, discard ¼ the bread)

2 pieces Canadian Bacon

With 1 packet ketchup   370   26

Bacon, Egg & Cheese Biscuit   348   27
(no Bacon, discard ½ the bread)

¾ Milk
With 1 packet ketchup: 351   30

Egg McMuffin   340   26
(no butter, no Canadian Bacon, extra Egg)

With 1 packet ketchup   350   29

Bacon, Egg & Cheese
McGriddle   365   23
(extra Cheese, discard ½ the bread)

With 1 packet ketchup   375   26

Bacon, Egg & Cheese
McGriddle   375   23
(extra Bacon, discard ½ the bread)

MEAL	CALORIES	NET CARBS
Egg McMuffin (no butter, extra cheese)	340	27
With 1 packet ketchup:	360	30
Scrambled Eggs	360	23
Canadian Bacon		
¾ Biscuit (no butter, no jelly)		
With 1 packet ketchup	370	26
Scrambled Eggs	350	30
Chocolate Milk		
With 1 packet ketchup	360	33
Scrambled Eggs	355	22
Hash Browns		
½ Milk		
With 1 packet ketchup	365	25
Scrambled Eggs	340	27
Cheese (on the eggs)		
Snack-Sized Fruit & Yogurt Parfait (discard Granola)		
With 1 packet ketchup	350	30
With Granola on Parfait	370	32

MEAL	CALORIES	NET CARBS
Scrambled Eggs	360	27
Bacon		
Snack-sized Fruit & Yogurt Parfait (discard Granola)		
With 1 packet ketchup	370	30
Egg McMuffin (extra cheese, with egg white only)	307	27
How to order: "Egg McMuffin, extra Cheese, with the egg white only."		
With 1 packet ketchup	317	30
Egg McMuffin (extra Cheese, extra Canadian Bacon, with egg white only)	327	27
How to Order: "Egg McMuffin, extra Cheese, extra Canadian Bacon, with the egg white only."		
With 1 packet ketchup	337	30
Egg McMuffin (no butter, extra Canadian Bacon)	310	26
With 1 packet ketchup	320	29

MEAL	CALORIES	NET CARBS
Egg McMuffin	360	27
Bacon		
With 1 packet ketchup	370	30

McDONALD'S Women   Lunch/Dinner

MEAL	CALORIES	NET CARBS
Cheeseburger (discard ½ the bread)	353	32
¾ Milk		
Cheeseburger (discard ½ the bread)	368	34
¾ Milk Side Salad (no dressing)		
Crispy Chicken Caesar Salad (no croutons)	360	27
½ packet Low-Fat Vinaigrette Dressing Apple Dippers (no dipping sauce)		
California Cobb Salad (no chicken)		
¾ Chocolate Milk	293	26

With ½ packet
Low-Fat Vinaigrette Dressing   313   28

Tip: You can order the salad with chicken
and save the chicken for snacks.

Extra Chicken = 3 Proteins.

6-piece Chicken McNuggets	348	27
¾ Milk		
With 1 packet ketchup	358	30
With ½ packet BBQ Sauce	371	32
With ½ packet Honey	371	33
With ½ packet Sweet-and-Sour Sauce	373	33

8 Chicken McNuggets	336	21

(order the 10-piece and eat 8; save 2 for snacks)

With 1 packet ketchup	346	24
With 2 packets ketchup	356	27
With ½ packet BBQ Sauce	359	26
With ½ packet Honey	359	27
With ½ packet Sweet-and-Sour Sauce	361	27

*Snacks: 2 McNuggets = 1 Snack (you can eat them
with 1 packet ketchup or 1 tsp. dipping
sauce)*

MEAL	CALORIES	NET CARBS

Fiesta Salad   340   31
(no chips, no sour cream, no cheese, no salsa)

Snack-Sized Fruit & Yogurt Parfait
(no granola)

Side Salad   305   29
(no croutons)

¾ Grilled Chicken for Salads (on the salad)
Chocolate-Dipped Cone (available at select
restaurants)

With ½ packet
Low-Fat Vinaigrette Dressing   325   31

Side Salad   265   26
(no croutons)

¾ Grilled Chicken for Salads (on the salad)
½ packet Low-Fat Vinaigrette Dressing
Cookie (any except peanut butter)

With Sugar Cookie	265	26
With Oatmeal Raisin Cookie	275	28
With Chocolate Chip Cookie	285	28

Snacks: Extra chicken = 1 Protein

MEAL	CALORIES	NET CARBS
Fiesta Salad	360	29
(no chips, no cheese, no sour cream, no salsa)		
Reduced-Fat Vanilla Ice Cream Cone		
With ½ packet salsa	375	32
Side Salad	275	29
(no croutons)		
¾ Grilled Chicken for Salads (on the salad)		
½ packet Low-Fat Vinaigrette Dressing		
Reduced-Fat Vanilla Ice Cream Cone		
With ½ packet Cobb Dressing	315	31
With ½ packet Caesar Dressing	350	29
Big 'N Tasty	365	23
(no mayo, discard *bottom* piece of bread)		
Double Cheeseburger	365	22
(order with just 1 piece of cheese, discard ½ bun)		
Tip: If sandwich comes with 2 pieces of cheese, discard 1.		
Fiesta Salad	355	23
(no tortilla strips, no sour cream)		
Apple Dippers (no dipping sauce)		

Meal	Calories	Net Carbs
¾ Chicken McGrill Sandwich (with mayo)	300	26
Side Salad (no croutons)	325	29
¾ Grilled Chicken for Salads (on salad) Small Fries		
With 1 packet ketchup	335	32
With ½ packet Low-Fat Vinaigrette Dressing (no ketchup)	345	31
With 1 packet ketchup + ½ packet Low-Fat Vinaigrette Dressing	355	34
Grilled Chicken Caesar Salad (no croutons, remove ½ the chicken—save for snacks)	300	32

½ packet Low-Fat Balsamic Vinaigrette
Dressing
Snack-Sized Fruit & Yogurt Parfait (discard
granola)

Snacks: Extra chicken = 2 Proteins

| Grilled Chicken Caesar Salad (no croutons, remove ½ the chicken—save for snacks) | 320 | 30 |

½ packet Low-Fat Balsamic Vinaigrette
Dressing
Reduced-Fat Vanilla Ice Cream Cone

Snacks: Extra chicken = 2 Proteins

Caesar Salad	290	30
(no chicken)		

Croutons (come with salad)
½ packet Low-Fat Balsamic Vinaigrette
Dressing
Milk

OLIVE GARDEN   Women   Lunch/Dinner

Tips:
- ✦ The Lunch Portion can be ordered for lunch or dinner.
- ✦ Hold the breadsticks.
- ✦ Don't add Parmesan cheese unless it's listed as part of the meal.

Condiments:
- ✦ Vinegar: up to 1 Tbsp.
- ✦ Lemon wedges: up to 2
- ✦ Chocolate Mint: 1

MEAL	CALORIES	NET CARBS
Chicken Giardino	348	30
(Lunch Portion, remove 7 pieces of pasta)		

1 plate of salad (no croutons, no dressing)
Use balsamic vinegar or lemon wedges for
dressing.

Chicken Giardino   360   36
(Lunch Portion, no salad or soup)

Shrimp Primavera   334   36
(Lunch Portion, no soup or salad, pasta and sauce on
the side)

Instructions: Add ½ of the pasta and sauce
to the shrimp and vegetables and eat them
together. Don't eat the other ½ of the pasta
and sauce.

½ Chicken Giardino   325   25
(Lunch Portion)

½ Minestrone Soup
12 grinds Parmesan Cheese (on the soup or pasta)
1 tsp. olive oil (in soup or pasta)

How to Order: "Chicken Giardino Lunch
Portion with Minestrone Soup." Ask for olive
oil, and a teaspoon. Makes 2 meals.

½ Chicken Giardino   302   21
(Lunch Portion)

1 plate Salad (no croutons, no dressing)
1 tsp. olive oil (on salad or pasta)
12 grinds Parmesan cheese (on the salad or pasta)

Optional: Use vinegar or lemon wedges for salad dressing.

How to Order: "Chicken Giardino Lunch Portion with salad, no croutons, no dressing." Ask for olive oil and vinegar (or lemon wedges), a teaspoon, and extra plates. Makes two meals.

OUTBACK STEAKHOUSE

Women   **Lunch/Dinner**

Tips:

   ✦ Hold the bread unless the meal includes it.

MEAL	CALORIES	NET CARBS
Chicken Caesar Salad with Small Chicken Portion (no croutons, no cheese, no dressing)	305	24

2 spoonfuls of Tangy Tomato Dressing (ordered on the side)
⅓ Loaf bread (eat with meal)
1 level spoonful butter on bread (ask for a spoon)

Remove ½ the chicken and save for snacks.

Snacks: Extra chicken = 3 Proteins

Meal	Calories	Net Carbs

Chicken Caesar Salad
with Small Chicken Portion   303   23
(no cheese, no dressing, croutons on the side)

2 spoonfuls of Tangy Tomato Dressing
(ordered on the side)

Remove ½ the chicken and save for snacks.
Use ½ of the croutons on your salad; don't
eat the other ½ of the croutons.

Snacks: Extra chicken = 3 Proteins

½ Chicken Caesar Salad
with Small Chicken Portion   341   28
(no cheese, no dressing)

1 spoonful Tangy Tomato Dressing
(on the side)
¼ Loaf bread (no butter)

Chicken Caesar Salad   307   21
with Small Chicken Portion (no croutons, no
cheese, dressing on the side)

1 spoonful Caesar or Ranch Dressing with 1
squeezed lemon wedge and pepper to taste
(on salad)
½ Loaf bread (eat with meal, no butter)

Eat 1/3 of the chicken with the salad. Save
the rest for snacks.

Snacks: Extra chicken = 4 Proteins

Shrimp Caesar Salad   286   22
(no cheese, no dressing, croutons on the side)

1 spoon Tangy Tomato Dressing (on the side)
2 lemon wedges (optional)

Instructions: Move shrimp aside. Squeeze
lemon wedges on salad. Add 1 spoonful of
dressing and pepper to taste. Mix with fork.
Add shrimp back to salad. Add 1/2 of the
croutons to the salad—don't eat the rest of
the croutons.

With 2 spoonfuls
Tangy Tomato Dressing   306   26

Shrimp Caesar Salad   335   22
(no croutons, no cheese, no dressing)

1 spoonful Caesar or Ranch Dressing
(on the side)
1/2 Loaf bread (no butter, eat bread with the
salad or after it—not before the meal)
2 lemon wedges

Instructions: Move shrimp aside. Squeeze
lemon wedges on salad. Add 1 spoonful of

dressing and pepper to taste. Mix with fork.
Add shrimp back to salad.

9 oz. Sirloin Dinner		
with Potato (dry)	308	30
No salad or soup.		

Eat ⅓ of the steak and ½ the potato.

Snacks: Extra steak = 6 Proteins
Extra baked potato = 3 Fruits

9 oz. Sirloin Dinner		
with Potato (dry)	292	24

House Salad (no croutons, no cheese, no
dressing)
Use lemon wedges for dressing

Eat ⅓ steak and ⅓ potato.

With 1 spoonful		
Tangy Tomato Dressing	312	29
With 1 spoonful		
Caesar or Ranch Dressing	369	25

Snacks: Extra steak = 6 Proteins
Extra baked potato = 4 Fruits

MEAL	CALORIES	NET CARBS

9 oz. Sirloin Dinner with Potato (dry) — 283 — 23

½ House Salad (no croutons, no cheese, no dressing)
Use lemon wedges for dressing

Eat ⅓ steak and ⅓ potato. Eat ½ the salad.

With 1 spoonful Tangy Tomato Dressing (on entire salad): 293 — 26

With 1 spoonful Caesar or Ranch Dressing (on entire salad) 322 — 26

Snacks: Extra steak (after 2 people have split the meal) = 3 Proteins
Extra baked potato = 2 Fruits

Atlantic Baked Salmon Dinner 366 — 28
(no sauce on the side, no butter on the vegetables)

⅔ Loaf bread (no butter, eat bread with meal)

Each person eats ⅓ salmon and ½ vegetables. Save the extra salmon for snacks. Each person eats ⅔ loaf bread (ask for a second loaf).

Snacks: Extra salmon = 3 Proteins

MEAL	CALORIES	NET CARBS

Shrimp Caesar Salad   298   31
(no croutons, no cheese, no dressing)

2 spoonfuls Tangy Tomato Dressing
(on the side)
½ Loaf bread (no butter, eat with the salad or after
it—not before the meal)

Optional: Move shrimp aside and squeeze 1 or 2
lemon wedges on the salad along with dressing. Add pepper to taste, and mix with fork.

Atlantic Baked Salmon Dinner 340   23
(no sauce on the side, no butter on the vegetables)

½ Loaf bread (no butter, eat with meal)

Eat ⅓ salmon. Save the rest for snacks.

Snacks: Extra salmon = 6 Proteins

PANDA EXPRESS Women   Lunch/Dinner

Tips:
+ Hold the chow mein and rice unless they are
  listed as part of the meal below.

Condiments:
+ Soy sauce: up to 1 packet (½ tbs.)

Meal	Calories	Net Carbs
Chicken with Mushrooms Chicken Egg Roll	320	23
Chicken with String Beans Chicken Egg Roll	360	27
Beef with Broccoli Chicken Egg Roll	340	26
Beef with String Beans Chicken Egg Roll	360	27
Spicy Chicken with Peanuts Veggie Spring Roll Mixed Vegetables	350	34
Black Pepper Chicken 2 orders Mixed Vegetables	320	22
Spicy Chicken with Peanuts ½ order Vegetable Chow Mein	365	33

PANERA BREAD   Women   Lunch/Dinner

Tips:

+ Hold the chips when ordering sandwiches.
+ Hold the side bread when ordering soups and salads.

Condiments:

+ Pickle: up to 1

MEAL	CALORIES	NET CARBS
½ Sandwich and Salad Combo:	358	27

½ Smoked Ham and Swiss Sandwich on Rye

½ Classic Cafe Salad (no dressing, no bread)

Squeeze 2 lemon wedges (from drink area) on salad for dressing.

MEAL	CALORIES	NET CARBS
½ Sandwich and Salad Combo:	328	30

Half Smoked Turkey Breast Sandwich on Sunflower Bread

Discard ¼ bread

½ Classic Cafe Salad (no dressing,
no bread)

Squeeze 2 lemon wedges on salad for
dressing (from drink area).

½ Smokehouse Turkey Breast Sandwich on Artisan Three-Cheese Bread	335	32

½ Sandwich and Salad Combo:	353	31

½ Chicken Salad Sandwich on
Nine-Grain Bread
½ Classic Cafe Salad (no dressing,
no bread)

Squeeze 2 lemon wedges (from drink area)
on salad for dressing.

½ Salad and Soup Combo:	285	32

½ Asian Sesame Chicken Salad
Vegetarian Black Bean Soup (no bread)

½ Salad and Soup Combo:	340	23

½ Grilled Chicken Caesar Salad
Low Fat Vegetarian Vegetable Garden Soup
(no bread)

Meal	Calories	Net Carbs
½ Portobello & Mozzarella Panini	325	34
½ Smoked Ham & Swiss on Rye	325	22
½ Salad and Soup Combo: ½ Grilled Chicken Caesar Salad Low-Fat Chicken Noodle Soup (no bread)	350	22

Pizza Hut   Women   Lunch/Dinner

Tips (Personal Pan Pizzas):
+ 1 Pizza = 2 Meals + 2 Snacks
+ ½ Slice = 1 Snack
+ At home, eat pizza with a dark green salad with vinegar or lemon juice.

Meal	Calories	Net Carbs
1½ slices Personal Pan Pizza, topped with:	315	27
Bacon Beef Extra Chicken		

MEAL	CALORIES	NET CARBS
1½ slices Personal Pan Pizza, topped with:	330	27
Beef Extra Chicken Extra Bacon		
1½ slices Personal Pan Pizza, topped with:	345	26
Pork Beef Extra Chicken		
1½ slices Personal Pan Pizza, topped with:	330	27
Extra Chicken Extra Beef		
1½ slices Personal Pan Pizza, topped with:	330	27
Extra Chicken Extra Cheese		

RED LOBSTER   Women   Lunch/Dinner

Tips:

+ The Lunch Portion can be ordered for lunch
  or dinner.

MEAL	CALORIES	NET CARBS
½ Tilapia (Lunch Portion) (no butter)	283	26

Double order of Vegetables (no butter)
1 Biscuit (no butter)
Garden Side Salad (no dressing, no croutons)

How to Order: "Fresh Tilapia Lunch Portion
broiled, grilled, or blackened with no butter,
Garden Side Salad with no croutons or
dressing, Double Vegetables with no butter,
lemon and vinegar on the side."

Snacks: Extra Fish = 2 Proteins

½ Red Snapper (Lunch Portion) (no butter)	300	26

Double order of Vegetables (no butter)
1 Biscuit (no butter)
Garden Side Salad (no dressing, no croutons)

How to Order: "Fresh Snapper Lunch Portion
broiled, grilled, or blackened with no butter,
Garden Side Salad with no croutons or

dressing, Double Vegetables with no butter, lemon and vinegar on the side."

Snacks: Extra Fish = 2 Proteins

½ Salmon (Lunch Portion)   291   22
(no butter)

Double order of Vegetables (no butter)
1 Biscuit (no butter)
Garden Side Salad (no dressing, no croutons)

How to Order: "Fresh Salmon Lunch Portion broiled, grilled, or blackened with no butter, Garden Side Salad with no croutons or dressing, Double Vegetables with no butter, and lemon and vinegar on the side."

Snacks: Extra Fish = 2 Proteins

½ Trout (Lunch Portion)   284   22
(no butter)

Double order of Vegetables (no butter)
1 Biscuit (no butter)
Garden Side Salad (no dressing, no croutons)

How to Order: "Fresh Trout Lunch Portion broiled, grilled, or blackened with no butter, Garden Side Salad with no croutons or dressing, Double Vegetables with no butter, and lemon and vinegar on the side."

Snacks: Extra Fish = 2 Proteins

MEAL	CALORIES	NET CARBS
½ Catfish (Lunch Portion) (no butter)	284	22

Double order of Vegetables (no butter)
1 Biscuit (no butter)
Garden Side Salad (no dressing, no croutons)

How to Order: "Fresh Catfish Lunch Portion broiled, grilled, or blackened with no butter, Garden Side Salad with no croutons or dressing, Double Vegetables with no butter, and lemon and vinegar on the side."

Snacks: Extra Fish = 2 Proteins

RUBIO'S FRESH MEXICAN GRILL
Women   **Lunch/Dinner**

Tips:
+ Hold the chips when ordering burritos.

Condiments:
+ Salsa: 1 to 2 containers at your discretion (see calories and net carbs below)
+ Lemon or lime wedges: up to 2
+ Onions and cilantro: up to 2 containers
+ Jalapeños: ½ whole (or ½ container sliced)

Salsa Calories and Net Carbs

Salsa	Calories/ Container	Net Carbs/ Container
Salsa Verde	5	½
Roasted Chipotle	10	1
Regular	15	1
Picante	30	1

Meal	Calories	Net Carbs
½ Baja Burrito (Carne Asada)	355	29
With 2 containers salsa	375	31
½ Baja Burrito (Chicken)	320	28
½ Baja Burrito (Carnitas)	330	30
½ Burrito (Mahi)	315	27
With ½ container salsa	320	28
3 Street Tacos (Carnitas)	330	27
With 2 containers salsa	350	29
2 Street Tacos (Carne Asada)	310	27
1 Street Taco (Carnitas)		

Meal	Calories	Net Carbs
Street Taco (Carne Asada)	320	27
2 Street Tacos (Carnitas) With 1 container salsa	330	28
Taco (Grilled Fish)	310	22
½ Grilled Grande Bowl (Chicken with Pinto Beans)	350	29
½ Grilled Grande Bowl (Chicken with Black Beans)	355	29
½ Grilled Grande Bowl (Carne Asada with Pinto Beans)	375	29
½ Grilled Chicken Chopped Salad	355	25
½ HealthMex Taco with Chicken		
Taco (Carne Asada)	330	30
Street Taco (Carnitas) With 1 container salsa	340	31
Taco (Carne Asada)	320	30
Street Taco (Carne Asada)		

SCHLOTZKY'S DELI   Women   Lunch/Dinner

Tips:

+ When available, squeeze 1 or 2 lemon wedges over your salad.

Cookies:

+ Meals containing a cookie were calculated using the Cookie with Real M&M's. Substituting other cookies adds the following calories and net carbohydrates to your meal.

Cookie	Calories Added to Meal	Net Carbs Added to Meal
Cookie with Real M&M's	0	0
Oatmeal Raisin	10	3
Chocolate Chip	20	3
Peanut Butter	30	0
Sugar	20	3
White Chocolate Macadamia Nut	30	2
Fudge Chocolate Chip	30	1
Cranberry Walnut Crunch	20	2
Golden Raisin Oatmeal	20	2
Triple Chocolate Chip	30	0

MEAL	CALORIES	NET CARBS
Chicken Caesar Salad (no croutons, no dressing)	344	25
¾ New York Creamstyle Cheesecake (discard the rest)		
With ¾ Cookies & Cream Cheesecake	359	29
Chicken Caesar Salad (no croutons, no dressing)	320	26
Schlotzky's Chips (any except Jalapeño)		
With ½ packet Light Italian Dressing	365	28
Chinese Chicken Salad (no chow mein noodles)	322	23
½ packet Sesame Ginger Vinaigrette Dressing Cup Chicken Gumbo Soup		
With Cup Beef Vegetable Soup	332	24
With Cup Vegetarian Vegetable Soup	350	26
½ Small Pastrami & Swiss Sandwich	293	26

Snacks: Extra meat and cheese = 2 Proteins

MEAL	CALORIES	NET CARBS
½ Small Pastrami Reuben	318	27
Snacks: Extra meat and cheese = 2 Proteins		
Chicken Caesar Salad (no croutons)	352	23
½ Old World Caesar Dressing Cup Ravioli Soup		
Chicken Caesar Salad (no croutons, no dressing)	316	24
½ Fudge Brownie Cake		
With ½ packet Light Italian Dressing	361	25
Smoked Turkey Chef's Salad (no croutons, no dressing)	339	30
Cookie (see page 152)		
Smoked Turkey Chef's Salad (no croutons, no dressing)	364	32
½ Fudge Brownie Cake		

MEAL	CALORIES	NET CARBS
½ Small Roast Beef & Cheese Sandwich	293	27

Snacks: Extra meat and cheese = 2 Proteins

½ Small Philly Sandwich	286	28

Snacks: Extra meat and cheese = 2 Proteins

Small Turkey Guacamole Sandwich (discard ½ the bread)	311	32

SUBWAY Women   Breakfast

MEAL	CALORIES	NET CARBS
Steak and Egg Sandwich with Cheddar Cheese (remove ¼ the bread)	348	25
Ham and Egg Sandwich with Cheddar Cheese (remove ¼ the bread)	328	25
Cheese and Egg Sandwich with Double Cheddar Cheese (remove ¼ the bread)	358	23

MEAL	CALORIES	NET CARBS
Steak and Egg Sandwich with Swiss Cheese (remove ¼ the bread)	338	25
Ham and Egg Sandwich with Swiss Cheese (remove ¼ the bread)	318	25
Cheese and Egg Sandwich with Double Swiss Cheese (remove ¼ the bread)	338	23
Steak and Egg Sandwich with Provolone Cheese (remove ¼ the bread)	338	25
Ham and Egg Sandwich with Provolone Cheese (remove ¼ the bread)	318	25
Cheese and Egg Sandwich with Double Provolone Cheese (remove ¼ the bread)	338	23

SUBWAY   Women   Lunch/Dinner

Sub Tips:

+ Hold the mayo and olive oil unless the meal
  says otherwise.
+ Bread: Any kind. Meals were calculated on
  white Italian bread. Calories and net carbs
  may vary slightly with other breads.
+ Cheese: Provolone, Swiss, or Cheddar (*not*
  American or Pepper Jack unless meal says
  otherwise).
+ Vegetables: Any

Condiments:

+ Mustard, vinegar, salt, and pepper: unlimited

Cookies:

+ Meals were calculated using Oatmeal Raisin
  Cookies. Other cookies will change the calories and net carbohydrates by the following
  amounts:

Cookies	Calories Added to Meal	Net Carbs Added to Meal
Chocolate Chip	8	1
Double Chocolate	8	1
M&M's	8	1
Chocolate Chunk	15	1
Peanut Butter	15	−3
White Macadamia Nut	15	−2
Sugar	23	0

MEAL	CALORIES	NET CARBS
Seafood & Crab Sub with Double Cheese (discard ½ the bread)	360	29
Veggie Delight with Double Cheese on Low-Carb Wrap	280	21
Cup Vegetarian Vegetable Soup		
Veggie Delight with Double Cheese on Low-Carb Wrap	340	22
Cup New England Clam Chowder		
Veggie Delight with Double Cheese on Low-Carb Wrap	298	25
¾ Lay's Original *Baked* Potato Chips		
Veggie Delight with Double Cheese on Low-Carb Wrap	360	26
Lay's Original *Baked* Potato Chips		
Mediterranean Chicken Salad (no dressing)	300	26
Side of Red Wine Vinaigrette Dressing (use all the dressing) Croutons (come with salad)		

Meal	Calories	Net Carbs
Cheese Steak Sub (discard ¼ the bread)	310	34
Seafood and Crab on a Low-Carb Wrap (no cheese)	352	21
Mediterranean Salad with Roast Beef (instead of chicken) ¾ Cookie (see page 152)	290	26
Turkey Sub with Cheese and Bacon (discard ¼ the bread)	325	34
Ham Sub with Cheese and Bacon (discard ¼ the bread)	335	34
Turkey & Ham Sub with Cheese (discard ¼ the bread)	290	34
Roast Beef Sub with Cheese (discard ¼ the bread)	290	33

Meal	Calories	Net Carbs
Subway Club Sub (discard ¼ the bread)	325	34
Add either Olive Oil Blend or Light Mayo		
Chicken Breast Sub (no cheese, discard ¼ the bread)	335	35
Add either Olive Oil Blend or Light Mayo		
Subway Melt (discard ½ the bread)	310	26
Dijon Horseradish Melt (discard ½ the bread)	370	36
Buffalo Chicken Sub (discard ½ the bread)	300	34
Turkey Breast, Ham & Bacon Melt (discard ¼ the bread)	340	35
Turkey Sub with Double Cheese (discard ¼ the bread)	330	34
Use 1 slice Pepper Jack Cheese and 1 slice either Swiss, Provolone, or Cheddar		

Meal	Calories	Net Carbs
Ham Sub with Double Cheese (discard ¼ the bread)	340	34

Use 1 slice Pepper Jack Cheese and 1 slice
either Swiss, Provolone, or Cheddar

TACO BELL   Women   Lunch/Dinner

Condiments:
+ Taco Sauce: unlimited

Meal	Calories	Net Carbs
Taco (Fresco Style) Chicken Soft Taco	340	30
Taco Chicken Soft Taco (Fresco Style)	340	28
Chicken Enchirito	350	28
Steak Enchirito	360	28
Chicken Soft Taco (Fresco Style) Pintos 'n Cheese	350	32

MEAL	CALORIES	NET CARBS
Taco Salad (no cheese, no shell, no sour cream)	330	21
Enchirito	380	29
Chicken Soft Taco	325	29
¾ Pintos 'n Cheese		

TGI FRIDAY'S　Women　Lunch/Dinner

MEAL	CALORIES	NET CARBS
Jack Daniel's Salmon	336	29

⅓ Salmon (no Jack Daniel's Sauce)
⅓ Baked Potato (dry)
Vegetables (no butter)
House Side Salad (no breadsticks, no
croutons, no cheese, no dressing)

Optional: Extra lemon wedges for salmon
and salad

Snacks: Extra salmon = 4 Proteins
Extra potato = 4 Fruits

MEAL	CALORIES	NET CARBS
Sirloin Steak	294	25

⅓ Steak

⅓ Baked Potato (dry) instead of mashed potatoes

House Side Salad (no cheese, no croutons, no dressing, no breadsticks)

Use lemon wedges or vinegar for salad dressing

Snacks: Extra steak = 4 Proteins
Extra potato = 4 Fruits

½ Chicken Caesar Salad	317	22

(no cheese, croutons on the side, chicken on the side, dressing on the side)

½ Breadstick (no butter)

Extra plate, lemon wedges, soup spoon.

How to Order: "Chicken Caesar Salad with no cheese, but with Croutons, chicken, and dressing on the side, 1 Breadstick, no butter, lemon wedges, a soup spoon, and an extra plate."

Instructions: Squeeze 2 lemon wedges on salad. Add 1 soup spoon of dressing and pepper to taste. Mix with fork. Divide salad evenly between 2 plates. Divide chicken and croutons evenly. Split the breadstick. Makes two meals.

MEAL	CALORIES	NET CARBS
Chicken Caesar Salad (no cheese, dressing on the side, croutons on the side)	367	23

1 soup spoon of Caesar Dressing
2 lemon wedges
pepper to taste

How to Order: "Chicken Caesar Salad, no
cheese, but with croutons and dressing on
the side, lemon wedges, and a soup spoon."

Use ⅔ croutons. Remove the 2 largest pieces
of chicken and save for snacks.

Suggestion: Before adding dressing
to the salad, remove some of
the lettuce to take home.

| Salad with ½ lettuce | 349 | 22 |

Snacks: Extra chicken = 2 Proteins

TOGO'S Women   Lunch/Dinner

Condiments:
+ Bread: any
+ Vegetables: any
+ Mustard: unlimited

MEAL	CALORIES	NET CARBS
#3 Turkey & Cheese (Regular, no dressing, discard ½ the bread, eat ¾ of the open-face sandwich)	288	28
½ #3 Turkey & Cheese (Large, no dressing, discard ½ the bread, eat ½ of the open-face sandwich). Makes 2 meals.	288	28
#2 Ham & Cheese (Regular, no dressing, discard ½ the bread, eat ¾ of the open-face sandwich)	309	29
½ #2 Ham & Cheese (Large, no dressing, discard ½ the bread, eat ½ of the open-face sandwich). Makes 2 meals.	309	29
#26 Ham & Turkey (Regular, no cheese, discard ½ the bread, eat ¾ of the open-face sandwich)	303	30
½ #26 Ham & Turkey (Large, no cheese, discard ½ the bread, eat ½ of the open-face sandwich). Makes 2 meals.	303	30

MEAL	CALORIES	NET CARBS
#16 Salami, Capicolla, Mortadella, Cotta (Regular, no provolone cheese, no oil, discard ½ the bread, eat ¾ of the open-face sandwich)	335	31
½ #16 Salami, Capicolla, Mortadella, Cotta (Large, no provolone cheese, no oil, discard ½ the bread, eat ½ of the open-face sandwich). Makes 2 meals.	335	31
#20 Albacore Tuna (Regular, no dressing, discard ½ the bread, eat ¾ of the open-face sandwich)	335	31
½ #20 Albacore Tuna (Large, no dressing, discard ½ the bread, eat ½ of the open-face sandwich). Makes 2 meals.	335	31

WENDY'S Women   Lunch/Dinner

MEAL	CALORIES	NET CARBS
Jr. Bacon Cheeseburger (no mayo)	350	31

MEAL	CALORIES	NET CARBS
Small Chili with Cheese	295	22
1 package crackers		
With 1 packet hot chili seasoning	300	24
With 2 packages crackers	320	27
Classic Single (no mayo, no cheese, discard ¼ the bread)	340	27
With mayo	370	28
¾ Grilled Chicken Sandwich with Cheese	278	26
Spring Mix Salad (no croutons)	330	28
½ packet Fat-Free French Style Dressing 1 Milk (8 oz., reduced fat)		
With ½ packet Reduced-Fat Creamy Ranch dressing	340	21
With ½ packet Low-Fat Honey Mustard	345	29
Mandarin Chicken Salad (no almonds—save for a snack)	334	31

Rice Noodles
⅓ packet Oriental Sesame Dressing

Classic Single	370	32
(no mayo, no bun)		

Jr. Frosty (or ½ Small Frosty)—be sure to ask which size they've given you because sometimes they give you a Small when you ask for a Junior.

Grilled Chicken Sandwich	330	34
(discard ½ the bread)		

Side Salad (no croutons)
½ packet Caesar Dressing

Kid's Hamburger	300	27
(discard ½ bread)		

Caesar Side Salad (no croutons)
½ packet Fat-Free French Style Dressing

With ½ packet Reduced-Fat Creamy Ranch Dressing	310	21

Small Chili	310	21
(no cheese)		

Side Salad (no croutons)
½ packet Caesar Dressing

With 1 packet hot chili
seasoning   315   23

WIENERSCHNITZEL   Women Lunch/Dinner

Tip:
+ Hamburgers contain more protein than hot
  dogs and may be more filling.

Condiments:
+ Mustard: unlimited
+ Kraut: unlimited

MEAL	CALORIES	NET CARBS
Original Hamburger	290	30
Deluxe Hamburger (no mayo)	290	30
Deluxe Hamburger with Chili (no mayo)	300	31
All-Beef Cheese Dog (use American Cheese, discard ¼ of the bun from each end—about up to where they hit the cheese)	330	16

MEAL	CALORIES	NET CARBS
All-Beef Cheese Dog with Relish (relish on the side, use American Cheese, discard ¼ of the bun from each end—about up to where they hit the cheese)	340	18
All-Beef Chili Cheese Dog (chili on the side, use American Cheese, discard ¼ of the bun from each end—about up to where they hit the cheese)	360	19
All-Beef Cheese Dog with American Cheese (discard ¼ of the bun from each end—about up to where they hit the cheese)	365	24
Original Hamburger with Chili	300	31

CHAPTER 4

Smart-Carb Men's Meals

A&W Men   Lunch/Dinner

MEAL	CALORIES	NET CARBS
3 Chicken Strips	500	30
Deluxe Hamburger (no dressing)	440	33
With ketchup and mustard	480	38
With dressing	500	36
Cheeseburger	500	40
Deluxe Cheeseburger (no dressing)	480	36
Hamburger	460	36

JUMBO MEALS

Meal	Calories	Net Carbs
Deluxe Bacon Cheeseburger (no dressing)	550	36
With ketchup and mustard	570	41
With dressing	600	40

APPLEBEE'S   Men   Lunch/Dinner

Meal	Calories	Net Carbs
Grilled Tilapia with Mango Salsa	431	40
2 soup spoons of Italian, Caesar, Blue Cheese, or Ranch Dressing on meal (order dressing on the side with a soup spoon)		
Teriyaki Shrimp Skewers	383	40
2 soup spoons of Italian, Caesar, Blue Cheese, or Ranch Dressing on meal (order dressing on the side with a soup spoon)		
Don't use the teriyaki dipping sauce.		
With ¼ teriyaki sauce	408	46

MEAL	CALORIES	NET CARBS

Sizzling Chicken Skillet   432   30
2 soup spoons of Ranch, Caesar, Blue Cheese or
Italian Dressing on the meal (order dressing on
the side with a soup spoon)

Don't eat the Ranch Dressing that comes with
the meal. Eat just 3 of the tortilla pieces.

**Half-Size Chicken
Caesar Salad**   478   39
(no Parmesan cheese, no croutons, no
dressing, no garlic toast)

1 soup spoon of Caesar, Ranch, Blue Cheese,
or Italian Dressing (order dressing on the
side with a soup spoon)
1 lemon wedge (order it on the side)
1 piece Berry Lemon Cheesecake

To the salad, add 1 soup spoon of dressing,
the juice from the lemon wedge, and black
pepper to taste. Mix with your fork.

Don't forget to have the Cheesecake for dessert.

**Half-Size Chicken
Caesar Salad**   478   48
(no Parmesan cheese, no croutons, no
dressing, no garlic toast)

1 soup spoon of Caesar, Ranch, Blue Cheese,
or Italian Dressing (order dressing on the
side with a soup spoon)
1 lemon wedge (order it on the side)
1 piece Chocolate Raspberry Layer Cake

To the salad, add 1 soup spoon of dressing,
the juice from the lemon wedge, and black
pepper to taste. Mix with your fork.

Don't forget to have the Chocolate Cake for
dessert.

ARBY'S Men   Lunch/Dinner

Condiments:
+ Ketchup: up to ½ packet

MEAL	CALORIES	NET CARBS
Roast Chicken Club Sandwich (no mayo)	390	37
French Dip Sub (no Au Jus Sauce)	440	40
With Au Jus Sauce	445	41
Martha's Vineyard Salad (no almonds)	470	33

Asian Sesame Dressing		
With Raspberry Vinaigrette		
Dressing	452	34
Save almonds for a snack.		

Asian Sesame Salad		
with Noodles and Almonds	465	30
¾ Asian Sesame Dressing		

Regular Roast Beef Sandwich	470	44
Milk (8 oz. reduced-fat)		

JUMBO MEALS

Meal	Calories	Net Carbs
Chicken Club Salad (no dressing)	580	34
½ Light Buttermilk Ranch Dressing		
Giant Roast Beef Sandwich	450	39
Chicken, Bacon 'N Swiss Sandwich	610	47
Chicken Cordon Bleu Sandwich	630	45

AU BON PAIN   Men   Breakfast

Tips:

✦ Bagel sandwiches were calculated on plain
  bagels. You can substitute other varieties.
  Calories and net carbohydrates may vary
  slightly.

✦ Adding a Small Cafe au Lait, Caffe Latte, or
  Cappuccino to a Woman's Meal (pg. 61) turns
  it into a Men's Meal.

MEAL	CALORIES	NET CARBS
Eggs with Provolone Cheese 428 ¾ Croissant	428	35
Eggs with ½ piece Cheddar Cheese and Bacon on Croissant 448 (discard ¼ croissant)	448	34
Egg on Bagel with Cheese & Bacon (discard ½ the bagel)	410	31
Eggs on Spinach and Cheese Croissant with ½ piece Cheddar cheese	435	34
Egg on Bagel with Cheese 405 (discard ¼ the bagel)	405	46

Egg and Bacon on a Spinach
and Cheese Croissant   430   31

Jumbo Meals

Meal	Calories	Net Carbs
Egg on Bagel with Cheese & Bacon (discard ¼ the bagel)	485	46

Au Bon Pain Men   Lunch/Dinner

Meal	Calories	Net Carbs
½ Roast Beef Sandwich with Cheddar and Swiss Cheese and Sundried Tomato Spread on Tomato Herb Bread	415	30
Grilled Chicken Ficelle Sandwich with Swiss Cheese	490	35
With Cheddar cheese	500	36
Roast Chicken Breast Sandwich with Sundried Tomato Spread on a Croissant (discard ¼ of the bread)	378	37

MEAL	CALORIES	NET CARBS
Ham Sandwich with Sundried Tomato Spread on a Croissant (discard ¼ of the bread)	408	33

BAJA FRESH   Men   Lunch/Dinner

Tips:
+ Hold the chips.

Condiments:
+ Salsa: Have any kind, up to the maximum specified in the meal.
+ Cilantro: unlimited
+ Chilis: up to 1
+ Lemon slices: up to 2

MEAL	CALORIES	NET CARBS
2 Steak Tacos	388	36
2 containers salsa		
Order with just 3 tortillas		
With up to 4 containers of salsa	414	41
½ Baja Chicken Burrito	410	32
With up to 4 containers of salsa	462	41

Meal	Calories	Net Carbs
Steak Taco Chicken Taco	410	45
½ Burrito Ultimo (Steak)	475	41
With 1 container of salsa	488	43
½ Burrito Ultimo (Chicken)	430	40
With 1 container of salsa	443	42
½ Enchiladas Verano ½ Guacamole (small side)	325	34
2 Chicken Tacos Guacamole (small side) 1 container salsa Order with just 3 tortillas	395	32
With up to 4 containers of salsa	434	39
½ Baja Steak Burrito	460	33
With up to 3 containers of salsa	499	40

MEAL	CALORIES	NET CARBS
Steak Taco	402	34
Charbroiled Fish Taco		
Order with just 3 tortillas		
With up to 4 containers of salsa	454	43

JUMBO MEALS

MEAL	CALORIES	NET CARBS
Steak Mini Tostadita (no sour cream)	630	55

BLIMPIE Men   Lunch/Dinner

Tips for Subs:
+ Bread: white or wheat
+ Cheese: any kind unless specified
+ Vegetables: any

MEAL	CALORIES	NET CARBS
Steak & Onion Melt	440	46
Golden Gate Gourmet Sandwich	400	38

Meal	Calories	Net Carbs
Grilled Chicken Sub with Mayo (no cheese, discard ¼ the bread)	363	38
Blimpie's Best Sub (discard ¼ the bread)	417	39
Ham & Cheese Sub (no mayo, no oil, discard ½ the bread)	378	38
With mayo	427	39
Turkey & Swiss Sub with extra Swiss Cheese (no mayo, no oil, discard ½ the bread)	445	36
Turkey Sub with Swiss and Provolone Cheese (no mayo, discard ½ the bread)	445	36

JUMBO MEALS

Meal	Calories	Net Carbs
Grilled Reuben Sandwich	630	48
Pastrami Sandwich (no mayo, no oil)	507	50

MEAL	CALORIES	NET CARBS
Turkey Sub with Extra Cheese (no mayo, no oil)	604	46
Ham Sub with Extra Cheese (no mayo, no oil)	616	48

BOSTON MARKET   Men   Lunch/Dinner

Condiments:
- ✦ Salt, pepper, Tabasco sauce: unlimited
- ✦ Lemon wedges: up to 2
- ✦ Ketchup: up to ½ soup spoon

MEAL	CALORIES	NET CARBS
One-Fourth Dark Chicken (remove skin)	450	33
Cornbread (no butter) 2 sides Steamed Vegetables		
How to Order: "One-Fourth Dark Chicken with 2 sides Steamed Vegetables." (Comes with Cornbread)		
Meatloaf	410	34
Fruit Steamed Vegetables		

How to Order: "Meatloaf with Fruit and
Steamed Vegetables, no Cornbread."

Ham	**390**	**33**

Butternut Squash
Steamed Vegetables

How to Order: "Ham with Butternut Squash
and Steamed Vegetables, no Cornbread."

Ham	**420**	**37**

Vegetable Rice Pilaf
Steamed Vegetables

How to Order: "Ham with Vegetable Rice
Pilaf and Steamed Vegetables, no
Cornbread."

Meatloaf	**470**	**42**

New Potatoes
Steamed Vegetables

How to Order: "Meatloaf with New Potatoes
and Steamed Vegetables, no Cornbread."

One-Fourth Dark Chicken	**430**	**33**

(remove skin)

Mashed Potatoes with Gravy
Steamed Vegetables

How to Order: "One-Fourth Dark Chicken with Mashed Potatoes and Gravy and Steamed Vegetables, no Cornbread."

One-Fourth Dark Chicken (remove skin)	420	30

Stuffing
Steamed Vegetables

How to Order: "One-Fourth Dark Chicken with Stuffing and Steamed Vegetables, no Cornbread."

One-Fourth Dark Chicken (remove skin)	410	35

Butternut Squash
Fruit

How to Order: "One-Fourth Dark Chicken with Butternut Squash and Fruit, no Cornbread."

½ One-Fourth White Chicken (with skin)	440	41

Steamed Vegetables
Green Beans
Cornbread (no butter)

How to Order: "One-Fourth White Chicken with Steamed Vegetables and Green Beans." (Comes with Cornbread)

Snacks: Extra chicken with skin = 3 Proteins

½ One-Fourth White Chicken 400 41
(with skin)

2 sides Steamed Vegetables
Cornbread (no butter)

How to Order: "One-Fourth White Chicken with 2 sides of Steamed Vegetables." (Comes with Cornbread)

Snacks: Extra chicken with skin = 3 Proteins

½ Turkey Breast 390 37

2 soup spoons Gravy
Chicken Noodle Soup
Stuffing

How to Order: "Turkey Breast with Chicken Noodle Soup and Stuffing, no Cornbread."

Snacks: Extra turkey = 3 Proteins

½ Turkey Breast 430 41

4 soup spoons Gravy
Chicken Noodle Soup
Mashed Potatoes

How to Order: "Turkey Breast with Chicken Noodle Soup and Mashed Potatoes, no Cornbread."

Snacks: Extra turkey = 3 Proteins

One-Fourth Dark Chicken (remove skin)	390	28

New Potatoes
Green Beans

How to Order: "One-Fourth Dark Chicken with New Potatoes and Green Beans, no Cornbread."

One-Fourth Dark Chicken (remove skin)	400	33

Corn
Steamed Vegetables

How to Order: "One-Fourth Dark Chicken with Corn and Steamed Vegetables, no Cornbread."

JUMBO MEALS

MEAL	CALORIES	NET CARBS
One-Fourth Dark Chicken (with skin)	630	45

Cornbread (no butter)
Steamed Vegetables
Green Bean Casserole

How to Order: "One-Fourth Dark Chicken
with Steamed Vegetables and Green Bean
Casserole." (Comes with Cornbread)

One-Fourth Dark Chicken (with skin)	620	42

Cornbread (no butter)
Steamed Vegetables
Green Beans

How to Order: "One-Fourth Dark Chicken
with Steamed Vegetables and Green Beans."
(Comes with Cornbread)

BURGER KING   Men   Breakfast

Tip:
 + If milk size is 10 oz., drink ¾ the amount
   listed in the meal.

MEAL	CALORIES	NET CARBS
Croissant with Ham, Egg, and Cheese	460	37

Meal	Calories	Net Carbs
Milk (8 oz.)		
With 1 packet ketchup	470	40
2 Egg Patties	400	28
2 containers Milk (8 oz.)		
With 1 packet ketchup	410	31
Croissant with Ham, Egg, and Cheese (extra ham, extra cheese)	450	28
1 packet ketchup		
Sourdough Breakfast Sandwich with Ham, Egg, and Cheese	480	40
Milk (8 oz.)		
With 1 packet ketchup	490	43

BURGER KING Men   Lunch/Dinner

Tip:

✦ If milk size is 10 oz., drink ¾ the amount
   listed in the meal.

Meal	Calories	Net Carbs
8 Chicken Tenders	440	32
Milk (8 oz.)		
With 1 packet ketchup	450	35
With 1 packet BBQ Sauce	475	31
With 1 packet Sweet-and-Sour Sauce	480	42
Whopper (no mayo, discard ¼ the bun)	478	38
Double Hamburger (no cheese)	440	29
BK Veggie Burger (no mayo, no bun)	445	42
BK Veggie Burger with Cheese (no mayo, no bun)		
Milk (8 oz.)		
Cheeseburger	450	42
Milk (8 oz.)		
Whopper Jr. with Cheese (no mayo)	450	42
Milk (8 oz.)		

MEAL	CALORIES	NET CARBS
Bacon Cheeseburger (discard ¼ the bread)	450	35
Milk (8 oz.)		

JUMBO MEALS

MEAL	CALORIES	NET CARBS
Whopper (no mayo)	540	48
Chicken Whopper	570	44
Hamburger	560	44
6-Piece Chicken Tenders		
With ½ packet BBQ Sauce	578	48
With ½ packet Sweet-and-Sour Sauce	580	49
Whopper Jr. (no mayo)	560	44
6-Piece Chicken Tenders		
With ½ packet BBQ Sauce	578	48
With ½ packet Sweet-and-Sour Sauce	580	49

CARL'S JR. Men Breakfast

MEAL	CALORIES	NET CARBS
Sourdough Breakfast Sandwich with Ham	450	38
With 1 packet ketchup	460	41
Sourdough Breakfast Sandwich with Bacon	470	37
With 1 packet ketchup	480	40
2 sides of Scrambled Eggs	473	30
¾ 10-oz. Orange Juice		
With 1 packet ketchup	483	33
With 2 packets ketchup	493	36
2 sides of Scrambled Eggs	500	36
Orange Juice (10 oz.)		
Scrambled Eggs	476	29
2 orders Swiss Cheese (on the eggs)		
2 orders Bacon (4 pieces)		
¾ 10-oz. Orange Juice		
1 packet ketchup		

Meal	Calories	Net Carbs
Side of Scrambled Eggs	510	35
Side of Swiss Cheese (on the eggs)		
Side of Bacon (2 pieces)		
Orange Juice (10 oz.)		

JUMBO MEALS

Meal	Calories	Net Carbs
Breakfast Burrito	560	36
Sourdough Breakfast Sandwich with Sausage	610	37

CARL'S JR.   Men   Lunch/Dinner

Meal	Calories	Net Carbs
Sourdough Bacon Burger (no cheese, no sauce, no butter on the bread)	450	36
With 1 packet ketchup	460	39
With butter on the bread	480	36
6-piece Chicken Stars	420	33
Milk (10 oz.)		

With 1 packet BBQ Sauce	470	44
With 1 packet Mustard Sauce	470	44
With 1 packet Sweet-and-Sour Sauce	470	45

3 Chicken Breast Strips	**453**	**32**
Garden Salad-to-Go		
Fat-Free Italian Dressing (as much or as little as you want)		
With 1 packet ketchup	463	35
With ½ packet BBQ Sauce	478	38
With ½ packet Mustard Sauce	478	38
With ½ packet Sweet-and-Sour Sauce	478	39

Famous Star Hamburger with Cheese	**461**	**38**
(no mayo, remove ¼ bread)		

Sourdough Cheeseburger	**465**	**37**
(no bacon, no sauce, no butter on bread)		
With 1 packet ketchup	475	40
With butter on the bread	495	37

Famous Star Hamburger with Cheese	**497**	**44**
(no mayo, no ketchup)		

Meal	Calories	Net Carbs
Famous Star Hamburger with Cheese (no mayo, no ketchup, remove ¼ the bread)	442	34

JUMBO MEALS

Meal	Calories	Net Carbs
Sourdough Bacon Cheeseburger	550	39
Charbroiled Santa Fe Chicken Sandwich	610	39

CHICK-FIL-A   Men   Lunch/Dinner

Meal	Calories	Net Carbs
Chicken Deluxe Sandwich	420	37
Chick-fil-A Sandwich	410	38
Chargrilled Chicken Breast (no bun)	440	29
Cheesecake		
With Strawberry Topping	460	37
With Blueberry Topping	470	38

MEAL	CALORIES	NET CARBS
Chicken Salad Sandwich	458	32
Side Salad (no croutons)		
½ packet Sunflower Seeds (comes with salad)		
½ packet Light Italian Dressing		
Southwest Chargrilled Chicken Salad (with sunflower seeds and tortilla strips)	455	30
Light Italian Dressing		

JUMBO MEALS

MEAL	CALORIES	NET CARBS
Chicken Sandwich	545	40
Side Salad		
½ packet Blue Cheese Dressing		
With ½ packet Caesar Dressing	550	40

CHILI'S Men   Lunch/Dinner*

MEAL	CALORIES	NET CARBS
½ Margarita Grilled Chicken Entrée	362	31

*Net carbohydrates were calculated using estimated dietary fiber based on similar ingredients, since dietary fiber information was not available at the time of this writing.

MEAL	CALORIES	NET CARBS
½ Margarita Grilled Tuna Entrée (no beans)	375	32
½ Chili's Cheesesteak Sandwich	367	32
½ piece Margarita Grilled Chicken Vegetables (no butter) Cinnamon Apples	428	36
Snacks: Extra chicken = 3 Proteins		
½ piece Margarita Grilled Chicken Vegetables Corn on the Cob	472	39
Snacks: Extra chicken = 3 Proteins		
½ piece Margarita Grilled Tuna Cinnamon Apples	467	44
Snacks: Extra fish = 4 Proteins		

MEAL	CALORIES	NET CARBS
½ piece Margarita Grilled Chicken	442	40
½ Fries ½ Vegetables (no butter)		
1 Bowl Chili	486	30
Dinner Salad (no cheese)		

How to Order: "Soup and Salad Combo with Chili. No cheese on the salad."

½ Turkey Sandwich (no Fries)	498	32
1 Cup Broccoli Cheese Soup		

How to Order: "Turkey Combo (no Fries) with Broccoli Cheese Soup"

1 Cup Chicken Enchilada Soup	440	31

Dinner Salad
2 soup spoons of Low-Fat Vinaigrette Dressing (on the side)

How to Order: "Soup and Salad Combo." Ask for the soup to come in a cup rather than a bowl. If it comes in a bowl, eat ½ of it.

JUMBO MEALS

MEAL	CALORIES	NET CARBS
Lettuce Wraps (use ½ the sauces that come with it)	598	39
Chicken Fajita Pita	501	44

CHURCH'S CHICKEN   Men   Lunch/Dinner

Tips:
+ No biscuits or butter with meals

Condiments:
+ Jalapeños: up to 1

MEAL	CALORIES	NET CARBS
Wing Macaroni & Cheese	460	30
2 Legs Mashed Potatoes with Gravy	460	30
Breast 2 pieces Corn on the Cob	478	34

Meal	Calories	Net Carbs
Wing	**490**	**34**
4 Jalapeño Cheese Bombers		
Breast	**440**	**30**
4 Jalapeño Cheese Bombers		
2 Krispy Tender Strips	**413**	**35**
1 BBQ Sauce		
Corn on the Cob		
With 1 Sweet-and-Sour Sauce		
(instead of BBQ Sauce):	**442**	**42**
1 Krispy Tender Strip	**457**	**39**
1 Leg		
2 orders Mashed Potatoes with Gravy		
2 Krispy Tender Strips	**395**	**33**
1 BBQ Sauce		
Coleslaw		
With 1 Sweet-and-Sour Sauce		
(instead of BBQ Sauce):	**397**	**34**

JUMBO MEALS

Meal	Calories	Net Carbs
1 Thigh	599	35
1 Leg		
Corn on the Cob		
Mashed Potatoes with Gravy		

DAIRY QUEEN   Men   Lunch/Dinner

Meal	Calories	Net Carbs
Grilled Chicken Salad	480	35
½ packet Fat-Free Ranch Dressing		
Chocolate Dilly Bar		
Grilled Chicken Sandwich	430	34
Side Salad		
½ packet Fat-Free Ranch Dressing		
Cheeseburger with Extra Cheese	480	39
Side Salad		
½ packet Fat-Free Ranch Dressing		
Grilled Chicken Salad	470	44
½ packet Fat-Free Ranch Dressing		
DQ Ice Cream Sandwich		

JUMBO MEALS

MEAL	CALORIES	NET CARBS
Grilled Chicken Salad	545	40
½ packet Blue Cheese Dressing		
DQ Ice Cream Sandwich		

DEL TACO Men   Lunch/Dinner

Tips:
+ If milk is 10 oz., drink ¾ of the amount specified in the meal.

MEAL	CALORIES	NET CARBS
Chicken Taco Del Carbon	490	37
2 Tacos		
Chicken Taco Del Carbon	430	20
Ultimate Taco		
Steak Taco Del Carbon	480	28
Ultimate Taco		

Meal	Calories	Net Carbs
Carnitas Taco	460	41
Taco		
Milk (8 oz. low-fat)		
Carnitas Burrito	440	38
Steak Taco Del Carbon	480	45
Beans 'n Cheese Cup		

JUMBO MEALS

Meal	Calories	Net Carbs
Deluxe Del Beef Burrito	590	41
Chicken Cheddar Quesadilla	580	39
Bacon Double Del Cheeseburger	610	31
Steak & Egg Burrito	580	38
Spicy Jack Chicken Quesadilla	570	38
Carnitas Burrito	600	48
Taco		

DENNY'S Men   Breakfast

Tips:

+ Syrup: use regular, *not* sugar-free
+ Eggs: order any style
+ Try Tabasco sauce on eggs

Condiments:

+ Salt, pepper, Tabasco sauce, mustard,
  vinegar: unlimited
+ Ketchup: up to 1 teaspoon
+ Half-and-Half: up to ⅓ container

MEAL	CALORIES	NET CARBS
1 Egg with Cheese (easy on the oil) Oatmeal (no sugar, no butter) Use the milk that comes with the oatmeal.	424	38
2 Eggs (easy on the oil) Oatmeal (no sugar, no butter) Use ½ the milk that comes with the oatmeal.	393	34
2 Eggbeaters with Cheese (on/in the Eggbeaters)	396	36

2 pieces Bacon
¾ Bagel

How to Order: "Original Grand Slam with
Eggbeaters, Cheese on the Eggbeaters, no
sausage, a bagel with cream cheese instead
of pancakes."

With ½ package cream cheese	446	37
With 1 package cream cheese	496	38

2 Eggbeaters	**477**	**42**

2 pieces Bacon
2 pieces Sausage
1 Pancake (no butter)
½ container syrup

How to Order: "Original Grand Slam with
Eggbeaters, Only 1 pancake, no butter."

2 Eggbeaters with Cheese	**479**	**33**
(on/in the Eggbeaters)		

2 pieces Bacon
1 order Hash Browns
½ English Muffin (no butter, no jelly)

How to Order: "The Triple Play with
Eggbeaters, Cheese on the Eggbeaters, no
sausage, no ham, English muffin, no
butter."

MEAL	CALORIES	NET CARBS
3 Eggbeaters	394	32
Cottage Cheese		
½ slice Apple Pie		

1 Egg	426	36
(easy on the oil)		
Ham		
Hash Browns		
½ English Muffin (no butter)		

How to Order: "The Triple Play, no bacon or sausage, only 1 egg, easy on the oil, 1 English muffin (no butter)."

With ½ package jelly	443	41

2 Eggs	432	40
(easy on the oil)		
Cheese on the eggs		
Fruit		
½ Bagel (no butter)		

How to Order: "2-Egg Value Breakfast. On the eggs, go easy on the oil. Fruit instead of Hash Browns. With ½ bagel (no butter)."

With ½ package cream cheese	482	41

MEAL	CALORIES	NET CARBS
1 Egg (easy on the oil)	452	38
Ham ½ Hash Browns Biscuit (no butter)		
How to Order: "The Triple Play, with just 1 egg, easy on the oil. No bacon, no sausage, 1 biscuit, no butter."		
1 Egg (easy on the oil)	367	39
1 piece of Bacon Ham Grits (no sugar, no butter)		
How to Order: "The Triple Play, with just 1 egg, easy on the oil. Just 1 piece of bacon, no sausage, no bread, 1 order of grits."		
With 3 tsp. milk	376	40

DENNY'S Men   Lunch

Tips:
+ Vegetable Beef Soup is currently offered on Saturday, Sunday, and Monday.
+ Senior meals are for guests 55 and older.

MEAL	CALORIES	NET CARBS
Seniors only	439	32
Senior Ham & Swiss on Rye (no Fries)		
Tomatoes instead of Fries	452	34
Seniors only	446	27
Senior Bacon Cheddar Burger (no mayo)		
Tomatoes (instead of Fries)	452	34
With Green Beans instead of Fries	473	28
Seniors only	490	32
Senior Tuna Salad Sandwich		
Cottage Cheese (instead of Fries)		
Ham Sandwich on Rye (no mayo, no cheese)	409	41
Chicken Noodle Soup		
How to Order: "Sandwich and Soup Combo, with Ham on Rye, no mayo, no cheese, and Chicken Noodle Soup."		
Ham Sandwich on Rye (no mayo, no cheese)	439	38

Side Salad (no croutons)

3 tsp. Ranch, Caesar or Blue Cheese Dressing

How to Order: "Sandwich and Salad Combo, with Ham on Rye, no mayo, no cheese. Salad with no croutons and dressing on the side."

With 3 tsp. Ranch Dressing	439	38
With 3 tsp. Caesar Dressing	441	38
With 3 tsp. Blue Cheese Dressing	456	38

Super Bird Sandwich (no mayo)	**492**	**35**

Tomatoes (instead of Fries)

Grilled Chicken Breast Salad (no cheese)—eat ¾ of the chicken	**384**	**34**

1 piece Garlic Toast (comes with salad)
Fruit Salad

Instructions: Have as many of the vegetables as you like, but eat ¾ of the chicken. Eat the salad dry, with vinegar, or with one of these dressings on the side:

With 3 tsp. Ranch Dressing	449	35

With 3 tsp. Caesar Dressing	451	35
With 3 tsp. Blue Cheese Dressing	466	35

Fried Chicken Strip Salad (no cheese, no bread)	405	33

Fat-Free Ranch Dressing

Turkey Breast Sandwich on Whole Wheat (no mayo)	450	36

Swiss Cheese (on the sandwich)
Side Salad (no croutons)
3 tsp. Ranch, Caesar, or Blue Cheese Dressing

Classic Burger (no mayo, no bun)	408	37

Fruit Salad (instead of Fries)
Raspberry Iced Tea

JUMBO MEALS

Make a Men's Meal a Jumbo Meal by adding a cup of Vegetable Beef Soup or a Small Milk.

DENNY'S Men   Dinner

Tips:

+ Vegetable Beef Soup is currently offered on
  Saturday, Sunday, and Monday.
+ Senior meals are for guests 55 and older.

MEAL	CALORIES	NET CARBS
Grilled Chicken Breast Dinner 403 (no bread)		36

Green Beans
Carrots
Side Salad (no croutons, no dressing)

Instructions: Eat the salad dry or with
vinegar or lemon wedges.

Sirloin Steak Dinner 478 (no bread)		25

Fruit
Tomatoes
Vegetable Beef Soup

Instead of Vegetable Beef Soup, you can
order a small milk and drink ⅔ of it.

Grilled Chicken Breast Dinner 434 (no bread)		31

Corn
Green Beans
Side Salad (no croutons)
½ packet French or Ranch Dressing (on
the side)

With ½ packet French Dressing	434	31
With ½ packet Ranch Dressing	447	29

Seniors Only	**363**	**34**

Senior Pot Roast Dinner (no bread)
Carrots
Corn
Chicken Noodle Soup

Seniors Only	**395**	**39**

Senior Chicken Strip Dinner (no bread)
Cottage Cheese
Tomatoes
Side Salad (no croutons)

Instructions: Eat the salad dry or with
vinegar or one of these dressings on the
side:

With 3 tsp. Low-Calorie Italian Dressing	403	41

With 3 tsp. French Dressing	458	41
Fried Shrimp Dinner (no bread)	395	39
Carrots		
Green Beans		
Marinara Sauce		

JUMBO MEALS

Make a Men's Meal a Jumbo Meal by adding a cup of Vegetable Beef Soup or a Small Milk.

EINSTEIN BROS. BAGELS   Men   Breakfast

Tips:

+ Sandwiches were calculated using plain bagels. You can substitute any other bagel (except for the Low-Carb or Power Bagel). Calories and net carbohydrates will vary slightly with other varieties.

+ Men can add a regular Latte or Capuccino (hot or iced) to any Women's Meal (p. 108) to make it the right size for a man.

MEAL	CALORIES	NET CARBS
Egg Frittata (discard ½ the bread)	430	38

MEAL	CALORIES	NET CARBS
Egg Frittata with American Cheese (discard ½ the bread)	500	39
Egg Frittata with Provolone Cheese (discard ½ the bread)	500	38
Egg Frittata with Sausage (discard ½ the bread)	500	38
"Naked" Ham and Egg Frittata (no bagel) Large Orange	440	30
"Naked" Ham and Egg Frittata (no bagel) Large Banana	445	31

JUMBO MEALS

MEAL	CALORIES	NET CARBS
Egg Frittata with Swiss Cheese (discard ¼ bagel)	590	56

MEAL	CALORIES	NET CARBS
Egg Frittata with American Cheese (discard ¼ bagel)	580	56
Egg Frittata with Sausage (discard ¼ bagel)	580	56
Egg Frittata with Cheddar Cheese (discard ¼ bagel)	590	55
Egg Frittata with Provolone Cheese (discard ¼ bagel)	580	55

EINSTEIN BROS. BAGELS
Men   **Lunch/Dinner**

Tips:

✦ When a meal says "no chips," you may be
   able to substitute a piece of fruit for the
   chips. However, don't eat the fruit with your
   meal. Save it for making snacks (page 32).

✦ Men can add a regular Latte or Capuccino
   (hot or iced) to any Women's Meal (p. 108) to
   make it the right size for a man.

Condiments:

✦ Pickles: up to 1

MEAL	CALORIES	NET CARBS
½ Albacore Tuna Sandwich on Artisan Wheat Bread	420	37
Cup Chicken Noodle Soup (no Lahvash Bread)		
½ Albacore Tuna Sandwich on Artisan Wheat Bread	430	34
Cup Broccoli Cheese Soup (no Lahvash Bread)		
½ Tasty Turkey Sandwich on Asiago Cheese Bagel (add cheddar or Swiss cheese)	505	34
½ Bros. Bistro Salad (no Lahvash Bread, no nuts, use ½ soup spoon of dressing on the side)		
½ Italian Chicken Panini	445	36
½ Bros. Bistro Salad (no Lahvash Bread, no nuts, use ½ soup spoon of dressing on the side)		
½ Roasted Turkey on Artisan Wheat	363	33
Cup Clam Chowder (no Lahvash Bread)		

MEAL	CALORIES	NET CARBS
½ Roasted Turkey on Artisan Wheat	393	42
Cup Tomato Bisque Soup (no Lahvash Bread)		
½ Roasted Turkey on Artisan Wheat	423	33
Cup Caribbean Clam Chowder (no Lahvash Bread)		
½ Cobbie Sandwich on Challah	505	34
½ Bros. Bistro Salad (no Lahvash Bread, no nuts, use ½ soup spoon of dressing on the side)		
½ Black Forest Ham Sandwich on Challah (extra cheese)	450	35
½ Bros. Bistro Salad (no Lahvash Bread, no nuts, use ½ soup spoon of dressing on the side)		
½ Albacore Tuna Sandwich on Artisan Wheat Bread	488	36
½ Chipotle Chicken Salad (no Lahvash Bread, use ½ soup spoon of dressing on the side)		

MEAL	CALORIES	NET CARBS
½ Albacore Tuna Sandwich on Artisan Wheat Bread	485	41
½ Bros. Bistro Salad (use ½ soup spoon of dressing on the side) 1/2 piece of Lahvash Bread (comes with the salad)		
Cup Turkey Chili	455	28
½ Chipotle Chicken Salad (no Lahvash Bread, use 1 soup spoon of dressing on the side)		
½ Ham & Cheese Panini	430	37
½ Bros. Bistro Salad (no Lahvash Bread, no nuts, use ½ soup spoon of dressing on the side)		

JUMBO MEALS

MEAL	CALORIES	NET CARBS
Chicken Chipotle Salad	630	31
Black Forest Ham on Challah (discard ¼ the bread, no chips)	545	49

MEAL	CALORIES	NET CARBS
½ Turkey Sandwich on Multigrain Bread	575	34
½ Asian Chicken Caesar Salad (no Lahvash Bread)		
½ Italian Chicken Panini	575	44
Cup Broccoli Cheddar Soup (no Lahvash Bread)		
½ Italian Chicken Panini	485	44
Cup Turkey Chili		

EL POLLO LOCO   Men   Lunch/Dinner

Condiments:
+ Salsa: 1 to 2 containers at your discretion (see calories and net carbs below)
+ Jalapeños: up to 1
+ Jalapeño sauce packets: up to 1
+ Lemon wedges: up to 2

Salsa	Calories (1 container)	Net Carbs (1 container)
House	6	1
Spicy Chipotle	7	1
Pico de Gallo	10	1
Avocado	20	1

Meal	Calories	Net Carbs
Tostada Salad (no shell)	360	28
With 1 container Pico de Gallo	380	30
With 1 container Avocado Salsa	400	30
Chicken Caesar Salad (no dressing)	429	30
Churro		
With 1 container Pico de Gallo	449	32
With 1 container Avocado Salsa	469	32
Chicken Taco al Carbon	372	32
Chicken Soft Taco		
With 1 container Pico de Gallo	392	34
With 1 container Avocado Salsa	412	34
Popcorn Chicken Corn Cobbette 2 orders Fresh Vegetables	447	36

JUMBO MEALS

Meal	Calories	Net Carbs
Chicken Quesadilla	593	48
Chicken Lover's Burrito	525	53

HARDEE'S Men   Breakfast

Meal	Calories	Net Carbs
Sunrise Croissant with Ham	430	28
Sunrise Croissant with Ham (extra American cheese)	480	29
Sunrise Croissant with Ham (extra Swiss cheese)	480	28
Sunrise Croissant with Bacon (extra American cheese)	500	29

JUMBO MEALS

Meal	Calories	Net Carbs
2 Tortilla Scramblers	620	36

HARDEE'S Men   Lunch/Dinner

Meal	Calories	Net Carbs
Slammer (no butter)	391	34
Fried Chicken Leg		
If Slammer is made with butter	406	34
Big Roast Beef Sandwich	470	36
Hot Ham & Cheese Sandwich	420	36
Slammer With Cheese	450	35
Fried Chicken Leg		
Slammer with Cheese	430	38
Milk (10 oz. low fat)		
2 Slammers	441	38
If Slammers are made with butter	471	38

JUMBO MEALS

MEAL	CALORIES	NET CARBS
Slammer Fried Chicken Thigh	570	49
2 Slammers with Cheese	560	40
Big Hot Ham 'n Cheese Sandwich	570	56
Charbroiled Chicken Sandwich	590	49

IN-N-OUT   Men   Lunch/Dinner

Condiments:

✦ Onions on burgers (order raw)

MEAL	CALORIES	NET CARBS
Double Meat Burger	480	39
Protein-Style Double Meat Burger (mustard and ketchup instead of spread)	458	31

½ container Fries

With 2 tsp. Ketchup	468	34
With 4 tsp. Ketchup	478	37

Cheeseburger	**480**	**36**

Double Meat Burger 400 41
(mustard and ketchup instead of spread)

Hamburger 442 41
(mustard & ketchup instead of spread,
discard ¼ the bun)

Protein-Style Hamburger (mustard and
ketchup instead of spread)

JUMBO MEALS

MEAL	CALORIES	NET CARBS
Cheeseburger (mustard and ketchup instead of spread) Protein-Style Burger (mustard and ketchup instead of Spread)	**560**	**42**
Double-Double (mustard and ketchup instead of spread)	**590**	**42**

JACK IN THE BOX   Men   Lunch/Dinner

MEAL	CALORIES	NET CARBS
Hamburger with Double Meat	460	29
5 Chicken Breast Pieces	405	34
1 packet BBQ Dipping Sauce		
With 1 packet Sweet-and-Sour Dipping Sauce	405	34
Sourdough Grilled Chicken Club Sandwich (no sauce)	445	34
Breakfast Jack	475	34
Ultimate Breakfast Sandwich (no egg, no bun)		
Breakfast Jack with Triple Ham	490	46
Milk (8 oz.)		
Deli Trio Pannido Sandwich (no sauce, remove ¼ the bread)	433	38

MEAL	CALORIES	NET CARBS
Asian Chicken Salad (no Wonton Strips, no Asian Dressing)	485	34
½ package Almonds (comes with salad)		
½ package Low-Fat Balsamic Vinaigrette Dressing		
Monster Taco		
Chicken Fajita Pita	380	34
Side Salad (no croutons, no dressing)		
With marinara sauce (for Chicken Fajita Pita)	395	37
With ½ package Low-Fat Balsamic Vinaigrette Dressing	400	37
With marinara sauce and ½ package Low-Fat Balsamic Vinaigrette Dressing	415	40
Southwest Chicken Salad	405	33
½ Spicy Corn Sticks		
¼ packet Low-Fat Balsamic Vinaigrette Dressing		

JUMBO MEALS

MEAL	CALORIES	NET CARBS
Roasted Turkey Sandwich	580	47
Ultimate Club Sandwich (no sauce)	530	47

MEAL	CALORIES	NET CARBS
Ham & Turkey Pannido	610	52
Philly Cheesesteak Sandwich	580	52

KFC   Men   Lunch/Dinner

Tips:
- ✦ Hold the biscuit unless it's listed with the meal below.
- ✦ Chicken and sides can be ordered à la carte.
- ✦ Small corn = 3 inches. Large corn = 5 ½ inches.

MEAL	CALORIES	NET CARBS
Drumstick (Original Recipe) 2 Orders Green Beans Biscuit (no butter)	430	33
Drumstick (Original Recipe) Drumstick (Extra Crispy) Biscuit (no butter)	490	32

MEAL	CALORIES	NET CARBS
Drumstick (Original Recipe)	480	30
Drumstick (Extra Crispy) Potato Salad		
3 Crispy Chicken Strips Small Corn	510	32
Drumstick (Extra Crispy) Wing (Original Recipe) 2 Small Corns (or 1 Large Corn)	450	30

JUMBO MEALS

MEAL	CALORIES	NET CARBS
Triple Crunch Sandwich (no sauce)	540	40
3 Chicken Strips with Biscuit (no butter)	590	40
Breast (Extra Crispy) Mashed Potatoes with Gravy	580	36

LONG JOHN SILVER'S Men Lunch/Dinner

Tips:

+ When ordering fish or chicken, ask for "no Fried Crumbs." Discard any that come with the meal.
+ Fish pieces are shaped like diamonds. Chicken pieces are smaller, with an irregular shape.

Condiments:

+ Ketchup: up to 1 packet (unless the meal says otherwise)
+ Cocktail sauce: up to 1 packet (unless the meal says otherwise)
+ Vinegar: unlimited

MEAL	CALORIES	NET CARBS
2 Chicken Pieces	500	41
Clam Chowder		
Shrimp & Seafood Salad (no dressing)	470	35
1 Chicken Piece		
With ½ packet Lite Italian Dressing	480	37
With ½ packet Fat-Free French Dressing	495	41

(Don't add ketchup or cocktail sauce when
using Fat-Free French Dressing.)

Crispy Chicken Salad	500	32
(no croutons, no fried crumbs, no dressing)		
Tip: Use malt vinegar for dressing.		

Shrimp & Seafood Salad	440	37
(no croutons, no Fried Crumbs, no dressing)		
2 Hushpuppies		
1 Chicken Piece		
With ½ packet Lite Italian		
Dressing	450	39
With ½ packet Fat-Free		
French Dressing	465	43

Shrimp & Seafood Salad	400	35
(no croutons, no Fried Crumbs, no dressing)		
Clam Chowder		
With ½ packet Lite Italian		
Dressing	410	37
With ½ packet Fat-Free		
French Dressing	425	41

Shrimp & Seafood Salad	460	38
(no croutons, no Fried Crumbs, no dressing)		
3 Cheesesticks		
1 Chicken Piece		

With ½ packet Lite Italian Dressing	470	39
With ½ packet Fat-Free French Dressing	485	43

2 Chicken Pieces	**510**	**27**
1 Fish Piece		

Shrimp & Seafood Salad	**480**	**31**
(no croutons, no Fried Crumbs, no dressing)		

2 Giant Shrimp
1 Chicken Piece

With ½ packet Lite Italian Dressing	490	33

(Don't add any sauces except vinegar when using Lite Italian Dressing.)

With 1 packet cocktail sauce (or ketchup)	497	35

Shrimp & Seafood Salad	**455**	**32**
(no croutons, no Fried Crumbs, no dressing)		

3 Battered Shrimp
3 Cheesesticks

With ½ packet Lite Italian Dressing	465	34

With 1 packet cocktail sauce (or ketchup)	472	36
With ½ packet Lite Italian Dressing and 1 packet cocktail sauce	482	37

JUMBO MEALS

MEAL	CALORIES	NET CARBS
Crispy Chicken Salad	590	40
½ packet Light Italian Dressing With ½ packet Fat-Free French Dressing	605	44

McDONALD'S   Men   Breakfast

MEAL	CALORIES	NET CARBS
Sausage McMuffin with Egg (no butter, no cheese)	490	30
2 pieces Canadian Bacon (on sandwich) 1 packet ketchup		
Sausage McMuffin with Egg (no butter, no cheese)	500	28
Bacon (on sandwich)		

MEAL	CALORIES	NET CARBS
Sausage McMuffin with Egg	450	31
Bacon, Egg & Cheese Biscuit	470	30
2 pieces Canadian Bacon (on sandwich)		
Bacon, Egg & Cheese Biscuit with Extra Cheese	500	31
Canadian Bacon		
Bacon, Egg & Cheese McGriddle	489	42
2 pieces Canadian Bacon		
Egg McMuffin (Extra Cheese, Extra Canadian Bacon)	370	27
With 1 packet ketchup	380	30
Scrambled Eggs	500	44
Canadian Bacon Hash Browns Chocolate Milk		
Bacon, Egg & Cheese Biscuit (discard ¼ the biscuit)	500	39
Milk		

Meal	Calories	Net Carbs
Scrambled Eggs	440	30
2 orders Bacon (4 pieces)		
English Muffin (no butter)		
1 packet ketchup		
With 2 packets ketchup	450	33
Egg McMuffin	410	27
(no butter, extra egg, extra cheese)		
With 1 packet ketchup	420	30
Egg McMuffin	380	30
(extra egg, extra Canadian Bacon)		
1 packet ketchup		
Scrambled Eggs	510	29
Sausage		
Canadian Bacon		
English Muffin (no butter)		
1 packet ketchup		
Scrambled Eggs	430	30
Cheese (on the eggs)		
Bacon		
English Muffin (no butter)		
Tip: Make into a sandwich.		
With 1 packet ketchup	440	33

MEAL	CALORIES	NET CARBS
Egg McMuffin	398	38
¾ Milk		
With 1 packet ketchup	408	41

JUMBO MEALS

MEAL	CALORIES	NET CARBS
2 Egg McMuffins (no butter)	580	52
With butter	600	52

Egg McMuffin (no butter)	580	48
Sausage Breakfast Burrito With butter	590	48

McDONALD'S Men   Lunch/Dinner

MEAL	CALORIES	NET CARBS
Quarter Pounder with Cheese	490	36
(order with only 1 piece of cheese; if sandwich comes with 2 pieces of cheese, take 1 off)		

MEAL	CALORIES	NET CARBS
Big 'N Tasty with Cheese (no mayo)	490	36
Chicken McGrill Sandwich (with mayo)	400	34
Big 'N Tasty with Cheese (no mayo, no bun) Reduced-Fat Vanilla Ice Cream Cone	460	28
Big 'N Tasty with Cheese (no mayo, no bun) Chocolate-Dipped Cone	510	32
Chicken McGrill Sandwich (no bun) Small Fries 1 packet Ketchup	450	31
Chicken McGrill Sandwich (with ketchup instead of mayo, no bun) Small Fries 2 packets Ketchup	370	37

MEAL	CALORIES	NET CARBS
10-Piece Chicken McNuggets	420	26
With 1 BBQ Sauce	465	36
With 1 Hot Mustard Sauce	480	33
With 1 Sweet-and-Sour Sauce	470	37

**Crispy Chicken Bacon
Ranch Salad**   420   27
(no croutons)

½ packet Low-Fat Balsamic Vinaigrette Dressing

Fiesta Salad   470   36
(no tortilla strips, no sour cream)

Reduced-Fat Vanilla Ice Cream Cone

Fiesta Salad   450   38
(no tortilla strips, no sour cream)

Snack-Sized Fruit & Yogurt Parfait (no granola)

Side Salad with Croutons   365   36

Grilled Chicken for Salads (on salad)
½ packet Low-Fat Balsamic Vinaigrette Dressing
Cookie (any except peanut butter)

MEAL	CALORIES	NET CARBS
Side Salad with Croutons	405	39
Grilled Chicken for Salads (on salad)		
½ packet Low-Fat Balsamic Vinaigrette Dressing		
Chocolate-Dipped Cone		
Side Salad with Croutons	405	40
Chicken for Salads (on salad)		
½ packet Cobb Dressing		
Reduced-Fat Vanilla Ice Cream Cone		
With ½ packet Ranch Dressing	420	40
With ½ packet Caesar Dressing	430	37
6-Piece Chicken McNuggets	455	35
Regular Hamburger (discard ½ the bun)		
With 1 packet ketchup	465	38
With ½ BBQ Sauce	479	40
With ½ Hot Mustard Sauce	485	38

JUMBO MEALS

MEAL	CALORIES	NET CARBS
Quarter Pounder with Cheese	540	36

MEAL	CALORIES	NET CARBS
Crispy Chicken Bacon Ranch Salad (no croutons)	590	44

½ packet Low-Fat Balsamic Vinaigrette Dressing
Small Fries

OLIVE GARDEN Men   Lunch/Dinner

Tips:
+ The Lunch Portion can be ordered for lunch or dinner.
+ Hold the breadsticks.
+ Don't add Parmesan cheese unless it's listed as part of the meal.

Condiments:
+ Vinegar: up to 1 Tbsp.
+ Lemon wedges: up to 2
+ Chocolate Mint: 1

MEAL	CALORIES	NET CARBS
Chicken Giardino (Lunch Portion)	414	39

1 plate of salad (no croutons, no dressing)

6 grates of cheese (on salad, on pasta, or split between them)

Optional: Use balsamic vinegar or lemon wedges for dressing.

Shrimp Primavera   416   40
(Lunch Portion, pasta and sauce on the side)

1 plate of salad (no croutons, no dressing)
12 grates of cheese (on salad, on pasta, or split between them)

Optional: Use balsamic vinegar or lemon wedges for dressing.

Instructions: Add ½ of the pasta and sauce to the shrimp and vegetables. Don't eat the remaining pasta and sauce.

Chicken Giardino   425   41
(Lunch Portion, remove 5 pieces of pasta)

Minestrone Soup

Shrimp Primavera   421   36
(Lunch Portion, with broccoli instead of pasta)

Minestrone Soup
1 tsp. olive oil (on the soup or pasta)

OUTBACK STEAKHOUSE

Men   **Lunch/Dinner**

Tips:

+ Hold the bread unless the meal includes it.

MEAL	CALORIES	NET CARBS
Shrimp Caesar Salad (no Parmesan, dressing on the side)	468	29
1 spoonful of Caesar or Ranch Dressing with 1 squeezed lemon wedge and pepper to taste		
Shrimp Caesar Salad (no dressing)	450	32
Squeezed lemon wedge and pepper to taste		
With 1 spoon Tangy Tomato Dressing	466	32
With 2 spoons Tangy Tomato Dressing	486	37
9 oz. Sirloin Dinner with Baked Potato (dry)	422	34
Dinner Side Salad (no cheese, no croutons, no dressing) Use lemon wedges and pepper for dressing		

Eat ½ steak and ½ potato. Save the rest for
another meal or for snacks.

With 1 spoon Tangy Tomato Dressing	442	39
With 1 spoon Caesar or Ranch Dressing	499	35

Snacks: Extra steak = 4 Proteins
Extra baked potato = 4 Fruits

9 oz. Sirloin Dinner with Baked Potato (dry)	394	30

Eat ½ steak and ½ potato. Save the rest for
another meal or for snacks.

Snacks: Extra steak = 4 Proteins
Extra baked potato = 4 Fruits

Chicken Caesar Salad with Small Chicken Portion (no Parmesan cheese, no dressing)	426	36

2 spoons Tangy Tomato Dressing (ordered
on the side)

Remove ½ chicken and save for snacks.

With 1 spoon Caesar or Ranch
Dressing and 2 lemon wedges

(instead of Tangy Tomato Dressing)	471	28

Snacks: Extra chicken = 3 Proteins

PANDA EXPRESS   Men   Lunch/Dinner

Tips:
+ Hold the chow mein and rice.

Condiments:
+ Soy sauce: up to 1 packet (½ Tbs.)

MEAL	CALORIES	NET CARBS
Spicy Chicken with Peanuts Chicken Egg Roll	390	31
Black Pepper Chicken String Beans with Fried Tofu 2 orders Mixed Vegetables	500	30
Chicken with Mushrooms String Beans with Fried Tofu 2 orders Mixed Vegetables	450	27
Chicken with String Beans String Beans with Fried Tofu 2 orders Mixed Vegetables	490	31

Meal	Calories	Net Carbs
Beef with Broccoli	470	30
String Beans with Fried Tofu		
2 orders Mixed Vegetables		
Beef with String Beans	490	24
Mixed Vegetables		
String Beans and Fried Tofu		
Beef with Broccoli	410	31
Black Pepper Chicken		
Veggie Spring Roll		
Beef with Broccoli	450	39
Chicken with Potato		
Veggie Spring Roll		
Beef with Broccoli	400	32
Beef with String Beans		
Veggie Spring Roll		
2 orders Beef with String Beans	420	33
Veggie Spring Roll		

MEAL	CALORIES	NET CARBS
Beef with String Beans	430	32
Black Pepper Chicken Veggie Spring Roll		

JUMBO MEALS

MEAL	CALORIES	NET CARBS
Chicken with Potato	500	37
Spicy Chicken with Peanuts Chicken Egg Roll		
String Beans with Fried Tofu	485	36
Spicy Chicken with Peanuts Chicken Egg Roll		
Chicken with String Beans	475	37
Spicy Chicken with Peanuts Chicken Egg Roll		

PANERA BREAD   Men   Lunch/Dinner

Tips:

+ Hold the chips when ordering sandwiches.

+ Hold the side bread when ordering soups
  and salads.
+ You can add a plain Cappuccino or a Caffe
  Latte to any Women's Meal (pg. 143) to make
  it the right size for a man.

Condiments:
+ Pickle: up to 1

MEAL	CALORIES	NET CARBS
Half Sandwich and Salad Combo 463 38 (no chips, no side bread) Half Frontega Chicken Panini Sandwich Half Classic Cafe Salad (no dressing) Squeeze 2 lemon wedges on salad for dressing (from drink area)	463	38
Smoked Turkey Breast Sandwich on Sourdough (no chips)	440	41
Asian Sesame Chicken Salad (no bread)	370	40
Half Sandwich and Salad Combo (no chips, no side bread)	398	31

½ Asiago Roast Beef Sandwich on Asiago
Cheese Demi
½ Classic Cafe Salad (no dressing)

Squeeze 2 lemon wedges on salad for
dressing (from drink area).

½ Sandwich and Salad Combo (no chips, no side bread)	463	38

½ Frontega Chicken Panini Sandwich on
Rosemary & Onion Focaccia
½ Classic Cafe Salad (no dressing)

Squeeze 2 lemon wedges on salad for
dressing (from drink area).

½ Salad and Soup Combo (no bread)	470	29

½ Grilled Chicken Caesar Salad
French Onion Soup

JUMBO MEALS

MEAL	CALORIES	NET CARBS
Chicken Salad Sandwich on 9-Grain Bread (discard ½ the bread)	565	40

MEAL	CALORIES	NET CARBS
Half-Sandwich and Soup Combo (no chips, no side bread)	520	46

½ Smokehouse Turkey Panini on Asiago
Focaccia
Low-Fat Vegetarian Black Bean Soup

MEAL	CALORIES	NET CARBS
Half-Sandwich and Soup Combo (no chips, no side bread)	625	47

Half-Italian Combo Sandwich
Chicken Noodle Soup

MEAL	CALORIES	NET CARBS
Half-Sandwich and Soup Combo (no chips, no side bread)	615	48

½ Italian Combo Sandwich
Low-Fat Vegetarian Garden Vegetable Soup

PIZZA HUT   Men   Lunch/Dinner

Tips (Personal Pan Pizzas):
  + 1 Pizza = 2 Meals
  + ½ Slice = 1 Snack

+ At home, eat pizza with a dark green salad
  with vinegar or lemon juice.

MEAL	CALORIES	NET CARBS
½ Personal Pan Pizza, topped with: Bacon Beef Extra Chicken	420	36
½ Personal Pan Pizza, topped with: Beef Extra Chicken Extra Bacon	440	36
½ Personal Pan Pizza, topped with: Pork Beef Extra Chicken	460	35
½ Personal Pan Pizza, topped with: Extra Chicken Extra Beef	440	36

MEAL	CALORIES	NET CARBS
½ Personal Pan Pizza, topped with: Extra Chicken Extra Cheese	440	36

JUMBO MEALS

MEAL	CALORIES	NET CARBS
2½ slices Personal Pan Pizza, topped with: Bacon Beef Extra Chicken	525	45
2½ slices Personal Pan Pizza, topped with: Beef Extra Chicken Extra Bacon	550	45
2½ slices Personal Pan Pizza, topped with: Pork Beef Extra Chicken	575	44

MEAL	CALORIES	NET CARBS
2½ slices Personal Pan Pizza, topped with:	550	45
Extra Chicken Extra Beef		

RED LOBSTER   Men   Lunch/Dinner

Tips:
+ The Lunch Portion can be ordered for lunch or dinner.

MEAL	CALORIES	NET CARBS
⅔ Tilapia (Lunch Portion)	397	34

Garden Side Salad (with 1 soup spoon of any kind of dressing on the side)
Double order Vegetables (no butter)
1 Cheddar Bay Biscuit (no butter)

How to Order: "Fresh Tilapia Lunch Portion broiled, grilled, or blackened with no butter, Garden Side Salad with dressing on the side (any kind), Double Vegetables with no butter, a spoon for the dressing."

Snacks: Extra fish = 1 Protein

MEAL	CALORIES	NET CARBS

⅔ Snapper (Lunch Portion)   419   34

Garden Side Salad (with 1 soup spoon of any
kind of dressing on the side)
Double order Vegetables (no butter)
1 Cheddar Bay Biscuit (no butter)

How to Order: "Fresh Snapper Lunch Portion
broiled, grilled, or blackened with no butter,
Garden Side Salad with dressing on the side
(any kind), Double Vegetables with no
butter, a spoon for the dressing."

Snacks: Extra fish = 2 Proteins

⅔ Salmon (Lunch Portion)   401   33

Garden Side Salad (no dressing)
Double order Vegetables (no butter)
1 Cheddar Bay Biscuit (no butter)

How to Order: "Fresh Salmon Lunch Portion
broiled, grilled, or blackened with no butter,
Garden Side Salad with no dressing, Double
Vegetables with no butter, lemon wedges
and vinegar on the side."

Snacks: Extra fish = 2 Proteins

MEAL	CALORIES	NET CARBS

⅔ Trout (Lunch Portion)   407   33

Garden Side Salad (no dressing)
Double order Vegetables (no butter)
1 Cheddar Bay Biscuit (no butter)

How to Order: "Fresh Trout Lunch Portion
broiled, grilled, or blackened with no butter,
Garden Side Salad with no dressing, Double
Vegetables with no butter, lemon
wedges/vinegar on the side."

Snacks: Extra fish = 1 Protein

¾ Catfish (Lunch Portion)   392   33

Garden Side Salad (no dressing)
Double order Vegetables (no butter)
1 Cheddar Bay Biscuit (no butter)

How to Order: "Fresh Catfish Lunch Portion
broiled, grilled, or blackened with no butter,
Garden Side Salad with no dressing, Double
Vegetables with no butter, lemon wedges
and vinegar on the side."

Snacks: Extra fish = 1 Protein

Note: Calories are based on a 5 oz. portion of fish before cooking
(4 oz. after cooking), and may vary depending on the actual portion served.

RUBIO'S FRESH MEXICAN GRILL

Men   **Lunch/Dinner**

Tips:

✦ Hold the chips when ordering burritos.

Condiments:

✦ Salsa: 1 to 2 containers at your discretion (see calories and net carbs below).
✦ Lemon or lime wedges: up to 2
✦ Onions and cilantro: up to 2 containers
✦ Jalapeños: ½ whole (½ container sliced)

Salsa Calories and Net Carbs

Salsa	Calories/ Container	Net Carbs/ Container
Salsa Verde	5	½
Roasted Chipotle	10	1
Regular	15	1
Picante	30	1

MEAL	CALORIES	NET CARBS
2 Tacos (Carne Asada, à la carte)	440	42
4 Street Tacos (Carnitas)	440	36

MEAL	CALORIES	NET CARBS
3 Street Tacos (Carnitas) 1 Street Taco (Carne Asada)	430	36
Taco (Carne Asada) 2 Street Tacos (Carnitas)	420	39
HealthMex Taco (Chicken) Street Taco (Carnitas) Street Taco (Carne Asada)	380	39
Taco (Carne Asada) 2 Street Tacos (Carne Asada)	420	39
Taco (Carne Asada) Street Taco (Carne Asada) Street Taco (Carnitas)	430	39
2 Street Tacos (Carnitas) 2 Street Tacos (Carne Asada)	420	36

MEAL	CALORIES	NET CARBS
3 Street Tacos (Carnitas) 1 Street Taco (Carne Asada)	430	36
Taco (Grilled Chicken) 2 Street Tacos (Carne Asada)	500	39
Taco (Grilled Fish) Street Taco (Carnitas)	420	31
Taco (Grilled Fish) Street Taco (Carne Asada)	410	31
HealthMex Taco (Chicken) 2 Street Tacos (Carnitas)	390	39
HealthMex Chicken Salad with Serrano Grape Dressing Small Guacamole (no chips)	400	30

JUMBO MEALS

Meal	Calories	Net Carbs
Taco (Grilled Chicken) 2 Street Tacos (Carne Asada)	500	39
Taco (Grilled Fish) Taco (Chicken)	610	43
Taco (Grilled Fish) Taco (Carne Asada)	540	43
HealthMex Chicken Salad with Serrano Grape Dressing Taco (Grilled Chicken)	530	48
HealthMex Chicken Salad with Serrano Grape Dressing Taco (Grilled Fish)	540	49

SCHLOTZKY'S DELI   Men   Lunch/Dinner

Tips:
+ When available, squeeze 1 or 2 lemon wedges over your salad.

Cookies:
+ Meals containing a cookie were calculated using the Cookie with Real M&M's. Other cookies will change the calories and net carbohydrates by the following amounts:

Cookie	Calories Added to Meal	Net Carbs Added to Meal
Cookie with Real M&M's	0	0
Oatmeal Raisin	10	3
Chocolate Chip	20	3
Peanut Butter	30	0
Sugar	20	3
White Chocolate Macadamia Nut	30	2
Fudge Chocolate Chip	30	1
Cranberry Walnut Crunch	20	2
Golden Raisin Oatmeal	20	2
Triple Chocolate Chip	30	0

Meal	Calories	Net Carbs
Chicken Caesar Salad (no croutons, no dressing)	371	34
Cup of Gourmet Vegetable Beef Soup Cookie (see page 257)		
With ½ packet Light Italian Dressing	436	39
Chicken Caesar Salad (no dressing)	376	29
Extra Mozzarella Cheese (ask for it on the salad) Garlic Cheese Croutons Cookie (see page 257)		
With ½ packet Light Italian Dressing	441	33
Chicken Caesar Salad (no dressing)	400	32
Extra Mozzarella Cheese (ask for it on the salad) Garlic Cheese Croutons Schlotzsky's Chips (any kind)		
With ½ packet Light Italian Dressing	445	34

MEAL	CALORIES	NET CARBS
Smoked Turkey Chef's Salad (no croutons, no dressing)	418	31
Extra Mozzarella Cheese (ask for it on the salad)		
Cookie (see above)		
With ½ packet Light Italian Dressing	483	36
Small Chicken Club Sandwich (discard ¼ the bread)	402	36
Salsa Chicken with Cheddar Wrap	460	41
Small Albacore Tuna Melt (discard ¼ the bread)	453	41
Small Ham & Cheese Original Sandwich (discard ¼ the bread)	456	41
Small Texas Schlotzky's Sandwich (discard ¼ the bread)	478	39
Smoked Turkey Chef's Salad (no croutons, no dressing)	451	32

Cup Broccoli Cheese with Florets Soup

With ½ packet
Light Italian Dressing   496   34

Smoked Turkey Chef's Salad   461   36
(no croutons)

Light Spicy Ranch Dressing
Cup Old-Fashioned Chicken Noodle Soup

JUMBO MEALS

MEAL	CALORIES	NET CARBS
Small Original Turkey Sandwich	583	51
Small Corned Beef Reuben	534	52
Small Fiesta Chicken Sandwich	577	50
Small Turkey & Bacon Club	571	50
Small Turkey Reuben	554	51

SUBWAY Men   Breakfast

MEAL	CALORIES	NET CARBS
Steak and Egg Sandwich with Double Swiss Cheese	430	32
Ham and Egg Sandwich with Swiss Cheese and Double Egg	470	33
Bacon and Egg Sandwich with Swiss Cheese and Double Egg	480	32
Steak and Egg Sandwich with Double Provolone Cheese	430	32
Ham and Egg Sandwich with Provolone Cheese and Double Egg	470	33
Bacon and Egg Sandwich with Provolone Cheese and Double Egg	480	32
Steak and Egg Sandwich with Double Cheddar Cheese	450	32

SUBWAY Men   Lunch/Dinner

Sub Tips:

+ Hold the mayo and olive oil unless meal says otherwise.
+ Bread: Any kind. Meals were calculated on White Italian. Calories and net carbs may vary slightly with other breads.
+ Cheese: Provolone, Swiss, or Cheddar (not American or Pepper Jack unless meal says otherwise).
+ Vegetables: Any

Condiments:

+ Mustard, vinegar, salt, and pepper: unlimited

Cookies

+ Meals were calculated using Oatmeal Raisin Cookies. Other cookies will change the calories and net carbohydrates by the following amounts:

Cookie	Calories Added to Meal	Net Carbs Added to Meal
Oatmeal Raisin	0	0
Chocolate Chip	10	1
Double Chocolate	10	1
M&M's	10	1
Chocolate Chunk	20	1
Peanut Butter	20	−4

White Chocolate		
Macadamia Nut	20	−2
Sugar	30	0

MEAL	CALORIES	NET CARBS
Mediterranean Chicken Salad 435 (dressing on the side) ½ Greek Dressing Croutons (come with salad) Lay's Original *Baked* Potato Chips		39
Mediterranean Chicken Salad 420 (no croutons, no dressing) Side Order of Swiss or Provolone Cheese (on the salad) Cookie (see page 262) Optional: Ask for vinegar on the salad.		34
Seafood & Crab on Low-Carb Wrap 462 (no cheese) Cup Clam Chowder		36
Seafood & Crab on Low-Carb Wrap 442 (no cheese) Cup Vegetable Beef Soup		33

Meal	Calories	Net Carbs
Seafood & Crab on Low-Carb Wrap (no cheese) Cup Cream of Broccoli Soup	482	34
Cold Cut Combo Sub with Double Cheese (discard ¼ the bread)	460	34
Sweet Onion Chicken Teriyaki Sub with Cheese (discard ¼ the bread) Add Olive Oil Blend or Light Mayo	465	44
Cheese Steak Sub with Double Cheese	440	43
Subway Melt Sub with Double Cheese	460	43
Roast Beef Sub with Double Meat (no cheese) Add Olive Oil Blend or Light Mayo		

Meal	Calories	Net Carbs
Dijon Horseradish Melt with Double Cheese (discard ¼ bread)	470	35
Turkey Breast, Ham & Bacon Melt with Double Cheese	430	43
Roast Beef Sub with Double Cheese	390	41
Mediterranean Chicken Sub	470	43
Savory Chicken Caesar Sub	490	42
Poblano Cheddar Turkey Sub with Double Cheese	370	42
BBQ Pulled Pork Sub (discard ¼ the bread)	390	42
Turkey and Cheese on Low-Carb Wrap Cookie (see above)	442	39
Turkey and Cheese on Low-Carb Wrap	417	34

Add either Olive Oil Blend or Light Mayo
Lay's Original *Baked* Potato Chips

With Doritos Nacho Cheesier *Baked* Chips	447	38
Turkey Sub with Double Cheese	380	42
Turkey & Ham Sub with Double Cheese	390	42
Ham Sub with Double Cheese	380	42

Ham Sub with Double Meat   395   43
(no cheese)

Add Olive Oil Blend or Light Mayo

Turkey Sub with Double Meat 385   43
(no cheese)

Add Olive Oil Blend or Light Mayo

Subway Club Sub with
Cheese   415   42

Add Olive Oil Blend or Light Mayo

Chicken Breast Sub with
Cheese   425   43

Add Olive Oil Blend or Light Mayo

MEAL	CALORIES	NET CARBS
Veggie Delite with Triple Cheese on Low-Carb Wrap	422	32
Lay's Original *Baked* Potato Chips		
Veggie Delite with Triple Cheese on Low-Carb Wrap	492	36
Cookie (see page 262)		

JUMBO MEALS

MEAL	CALORIES	NET CARBS
Ham Sub with Cheese (extra meat, extra cheese)	495	43
Add Olive Oil Blend or Light Mayo		
Roast Beef Sub with Cheese (extra meat, extra cheese)	505	42
Add Olive Oil Blend or Light Mayo		
Turkey Sub with Cheese (extra meat, extra cheese)	485	44
Add Olive Oil Blend or Light Mayo		

TACO BELL   Men   Lunch/Dinner

Condiments:
+ Taco Sauce: unlimited

MEAL	CALORIES	NET CARBS
2 Chicken Soft Tacos	380	37
Taco Salad (no sour cream, discard ⅔ of the shell)	484	33
Taco Salad (no cheese, no shell, no sour cream) Taco (Fresco Style)	480	32
Chicken Soft Taco Steak Soft Taco	470	39
Chicken Soft Taco (Fresco Style) Taco (Fresco Style) Pintos 'n Cheese	500	43
Taco Taco (Fresco Style) Pintos 'n Cheese	500	25

JUMBO MEALS

MEAL	CALORIES	NET CARBS
Chicken Enchirito Taco	520	38
2 Tacos (Fresco Style) 2 Chicken Soft Tacos	530	49

TGI FRIDAY'S Men   Lunch/Dinner

MEAL	CALORIES	NET CARBS
½ Sirloin Steak ½ Plain Baked Potato (no butter, no sour cream) House Side Salad (no cheese, no croutons, no dressing, no Breadstick) Use lemon wedges or vinegar for salad dressing *Snacks: Extra steak = 3 Proteins* *Extra potato = 3 Fruits*	424	36
Chicken Caesar Salad (no cheese, dressing on the side) 1 soup spoon Caesar Dressing and 2 lemon wedges and pepper to taste	467	31

MEAL	CALORIES	NET CARBS

How to Order: "Chicken Caesar Salad, no cheese, dressing on the side, lemon wedges, and a soup spoon."

Instructions: Remove 2 largest pieces of chicken and save for snacks. Move croutons and remaining chicken to the sides of plate. Squeeze lemon wedges over salad. Add 1 soup spoon of dressing and pepper to taste. Mix with fork.

Suggestion: The salad comes with a lot of lettuce. Before adding dressing to the salad, remove some of the lettuce to take home.

Salad with ½ lettuce	449	30

Snacks: Extra chicken = 2 Proteins

½ Jack Daniel's Salmon	472	40

(no Jack Daniel's Sauce)

½ Baked Potato (dry)
Vegetables (no butter)
House Side Salad (no cheese, no croutons, no dressing, no breadstick)

Optional: Lemon wedges and/or vinegar for salad and salmon

Snacks: Extra salmon = 3 Proteins
Extra potato = 3 Fruits

TOGO'S Men   Lunch/Dinner

Condiments:
+ Bread: any
+ Vegetables: any
+ Mustard: unlimited

MEAL	CALORIES	NET CARBS
#3 Turkey & Cheese (Regular, no dressing, discard ½ the bread)	384	37
#2 Ham & Cheese (Regular, no dressing, discard ½ the bread)	412	39
#26 Ham & Turkey (Regular, no cheese, discard ½ the bread)	404	40
#16 Salami, Capicolla, Mortadella, Cotta (Regular, no provolone cheese, no oil, discard ½ the bread)	446	41
#20 Albacore Tuna (Regular, no dressing, discard ½ the bread)	447	41

JUMBO MEALS

MEAL	CALORIES	NET CARBS
#23 Italian Dry Salami & Cheese (Regular, no dressing, discard ½ the bread)	550	44
With dressing	607	46
#6 Meatball Sub (Regular, discard ½ the bread)	540	46
#26 Turkey & Ham with Cheese (Regular, discard ½ the bread)	503	44

WENDY'S Men   Lunch/Dinner

MEAL	CALORIES	NET CARBS
Chicken Club Sandwich (no mayo)	440	43
With mayo	470	44

MEAL	CALORIES	NET CARBS
Chicken Breast Fillet Sandwich (no mayo)	400	43
With mayo	430	44
Spicy Chicken Sandwich (no mayo)	400	43
With mayo	430	44
Classic Single (no cheese, no mayo)	380	34
With mayo	410	35
Mandarin Chicken Salad with Rice Noodles and Almonds (use 1/3 packet Oriental Sesame Dressing)	464	33
Classic Single with Cheese (no mayo, no bun)	440	32

Jr. Frosty (or 1/2 Small Frosty)—be sure to ask which size they've given you because sometimes they give you a Small when you ask for a Junior.

MEAL	CALORIES	NET CARBS
Grilled Chicken Sandwich	399	42
Side Salad		
⅓ packet House Vinaigrette Dressing		
With ½ packet Caesar Dressing	410	39
Small Chili with Double Cheese	390	28
2 packages crackers		
With 1 packet Hot Chili Seasoning	395	30
With 3 packages crackers	415	35
Small Chili with Cheese	445	37
2 packages crackers		
Caesar Side Salad (no croutons)		
½ Low-Fat Honey-Mustard Dressing		
With 1 packet Hot Chili seasoning	450	39
Taco Supremo Salad with Salsa (no sour cream, no chips)	390	27

With 1 packet Hot Chili seasoning	395	29
With sour cream	450	29
Classic Single with Cheese (no mayo)	450	35
With mayo	480	36
Large Chili with Cheese 1 package crackers	395	30
With 1 packet Hot Chili Seasoning	400	32
Grilled Chicken Sandwich with Cheese	370	35

JUMBO MEALS

MEAL	CALORIES	NET CARBS
Big Bacon Classic (no mayo)	550	42

WIENERSCHNITZEL   Men   Lunch/Dinner

Tip:
+ Hamburgers contain more protein than hot
  dogs and may be more filling.

Condiments:
+ Mustard: unlimited
+ Kraut: unlimited

MEAL	CALORIES	NET CARBS
Deluxe Cheeseburger with Extra Cheese (no mayo)	470	30
All Beef Chili Cheese Dog (Cheddar Cheese)	490	33
All-Beef Chili Cheese Dog with Relish (Cheddar Cheese)	500	35
All-Beef Cheese Dog (Cheddar Cheese)	460	31
All-Beef Cheese Dog with Relish (Cheddar Cheese)	470	33

MEAL	CALORIES	NET CARBS
All-Beef Chili Cheese Dog with Extra Cheese (American Cheese)	480	32
All-Beef Chili Cheese Dog with Extra Cheese with Relish (American Cheese)	490	34
Chili Cheeseburger with Extra Cheese	400	31

JUMBO MEALS

MEAL	CALORIES	NET CARBS
Hamburger	570	46
All-Beef Mustard Dog (discard ½ the bread)		

How *Smart-Carb Guide* Meals Are Calculated

Smart-Carb Guide calculations and portion sizes are based on those used in *The Zone* by Barry Sears, Ph.D. (ReganBooks, 1995).

The nutritional values used to calculate *Smart-Carb Guide* meals come from the individual restaurants, which publish test results from independent laboratories. Most nutritional values can be found on the restaurants' websites. When information was not available online or at franchises, it was obtained by contacting the restaurants' corporate offices directly. Data used in this edition of *The Smart-Carb Guide* is based on nutritional information made publicly available as of this writing.

When nutritional data was incomplete or unavailable, meals at restaurants were sampled and the meal components were weighed and recorded. Nutritional data from the U.S. Department of Agriculture (www.nal.usda.gov/fnic/foodcomp/search) was used calculate nutrients in meal and snack components. When the amount of an ingredient was unknown (such as in salad dressings), nutritional information for standard commercial varieties was substituted.

The 40-30-30 Formula

The following method was used to obtain ratios consistent with the 40-30-30 dietary formula used in *Enter the Zone*:

1. Obtain grams protein, total carbohydrates, and fiber for a meal.
2. Subtract fiber from total carbohydrates to yield net carbohydrates:

   total carbohydrates − fiber =
   net carbohydrates

3. Divide protein by net carbohydrates to yield the protein-carbohydrate ratio:

   protein ÷ net carbohydrates =
   protein-carbohydrate ratio

4. The protein-carbohydrate ratio was considered acceptable if it was between 0.6 and 1.0.
5. Obtain calories from fat and total calories for the meal.

6. Divide calories from fat by total calories and multiply by 100 to yield percent of fat:

   calories from fat ÷ total calories × 100 =
   percent of fat

7. The percent of fat was considered acceptable if it was 25 percent or greater. Most *Smart-Carb Guide* meals contain at least 30 percent.

PROTEIN

Smart-Carb Guide meals contain the following amounts of protein:

Meal Type	Average Protein (g)	Range of Protein (g)
Women's	21	18½–23½
Men's	27	24½–29½
Jumbo	35	32½–37½

CALORIES

Maximum calories for meals were set as follows:

Meal Type	Maximum Calories
Women's	375
Men's	500
Jumbo	625

EXCEPTIONS

A limited number of meals that fell outside the limits were included at the author's discretion if, upon testing, they were found to be satisfying for four to six hours.

SNACKS

The U.S. Department of Agriculture nutritional values were used to design snacks that balance protein and carbohydrates and contain approximately 100 calories.

APPENDIX B

. . . . . .

Determining
Fruit Size

To learn the size of your fruit, weigh it on a food scale, either at home or at the grocery store. Find the weight of your fruit in the chart below to learn whether it's small, medium, or large.

Smart-Carb Tip: Use Your Fist!

Notice whether the fruit is smaller than, the same size as, or bigger than your fist. If it's small like an apricot, notice whether it's ⅓ or ½ the size of your fist. In the future, use your fist instead of a scale!

Fruit Sizes and Weights*

Fruit	Size	Ounces	Pounds
Apple	Small	4–5½	.025–0.34
Apple	Medium	6–7½	038–0.47
Apricot	Large	3–3½	0.19–0.22
Banana (with peel)	Small	3½–4½	0.22–0.28
Banana (with peel)	Medium	5–7	0.31–0.44
Cantaloupe	1 cup	5½	0.34
Grapes	1 cup	5½	0.34
Honeydew	1 cup	5½	0.34
Nectarine	Small	4½–5½	0.28–0.34
Nectarine	Medium	6–7	0.38–0.44
Nectarine	Large	7½–8½	0.47–0.53
Orange (with peel)	Small	3½–6	0.22–0.38
Orange (with peel)	Medium	6½–10	0.41–0.63
Orange (with peel)	Large	10½–15	0.66–0.94
Peach	Small	4½–5 ½	0.28–0.34

Peach	Medium	6–7	0.38–0.44
Peach	Large	7½–8½	0.47–0.53
Pear	Small	4–5½	0.25–0.34
Pear	Medium	6–7½	0.38–0.47
Plum	Small	2½–3	0.16–0.19
Plum	Medium	3½–4	0.22–0.25
Plum	Large	4½–5	0.28–0.31
Strawberries	1 cup	5½	0.34

Smart-Carb Tip: Using Scales at Grocery Stores

1. Use ounces for nondigital scales. Use pounds for digital scales.
2. Most nondigital scales measure in ounces. But if a scale is labeled "⅒ pound" or "0.1 pound," don't use it because it won't be compatible with the chart below.
3. If the pointer doesn't line up with zero, vary your position until it *looks* like the pointer lines up with zero. Keep looking at the pointer while you weigh your fruit.

*Fruit sizes used in this book are the author's interpretation of commonly perceived sizes and are not necessarily the same as U.S. Department of Agriculture classifications.

Index

After-lunch coma, 12
Animal foods, 17–18
Applebee's, 56–60, 172–74
Arby's, 60–61, 174–75
Atkins Diet, 21
Au Bon Pain, 61–63, 176–78
A&W, 55–56, 171–72

Bacon
  Big Classic Meal, 275
  and Double Egg Sandwich
    with Cheese, 261
  Egg & Cheese Biscuit,
    125–26, 232
  Egg & Cheese McGriddle,
    126, 232
  on Sandwich, 231
  Side, 76–77
  Sourdough Sandwich, 76,
    191
  Sunrise Croissant, 220
Baja Fresh, 64–67, 178–80
Balanced meal, 4–5
  health benefits of, 6–7

nutritional components of,
  3–4
Beans, 45
Beef
  with Broccoli, 142, 243
  with String Beans, 142,
    243–44
Blimpie, 67–68, 180–82
Blood sugar, 12, 16
Boca Burger, 99
Boston Market, 68–71,
  182–87
Breakfast Jack, 120, 224
  with Triple Ham, 224
Burger King, 72–75, 187–90
Burrito
  Baja Carne Asada, 150
  Baja Carnitas, 150
  Baja Chicken, 65, 150, 178
  Baja Steak, 179
  Breakfast, 192
  Carnitas, 87, 202
  Chicken Lover's, 112, 220
  Del Beef, 86

Del Beef Deluxe, 202
Mahi, 150
Steak & Egg, 202
Ultimo (Chicken), 179

Calories, 26
Carbohydrates, 7–9, 11–12
Carl's Jr., 76–79, 191–94
Caveman Dinner, 9–10
Cheese
    and Egg Sandwich with
        Double Cheese, 155–156
Cheeseburger
    A&W, 56, 171
    A&W Deluxe, 56, 171
    Bacon, 74, 190
    Bacon Double Del, 202
    Burger King, 62, 189
    Chili with Extra Cheese,
        277
    Dairy Queen, 85
    Deluxe Bacon, 172
    Deluxe with Extra Cheese,
        276
    Double, 85, 132
    with Extra Cheese, 200
    In-N-Out, 118, 223
    Jack in the Box, 118
    Jr. Bacon, 166
    McDonald's, 129
    Sourdough, 193
    Sourdough Bacon, 194
Cheesecake, 153, 194
Cheese dog
    All-Beef, 169, 276
    All-Beef Chili, 170, 276
    All-Beef Chili with Extra
        Cheese, 277
    All-Beef Chili with Relish,
        276
    All-Beef Chili with Relish
        and Extra Cheese,
        277

All-Beef with American
    Cheese, 170
All-Beef with Relish, 170,
    276
Cheesesteak Sandwich, 196
Chicken
    Bacon 'N Swiss Sandwich,
        175
    Big Sandwich, 116
    Black Pepper, 142, 242,
        244
    Breast, 199
    Breast, Extra Crispy, 227
    Breast, Flame-Grilled,
        111–13
    Breast Fillet Sandwich, 273
    Breast Meal, 84, 198–99
    Breast Pieces (5), 224
    Breast Strips, 193
    Carver Sandwich, 70
    Charbroiled Sandwich, 222
    Charbroiled Sandwich with
        Mayo, 116
    Charbroiled Santa Fe
        Sandwich, 77, 194
    Chick-fil-A Sandwich,
        79–80
    Club Sandwich, 272
    Cordon Bleu Sandwich,
        175
    Dark, 71
    Deluxe Sandwich, 61, 80,
        194
    Drumstick (Extra Crispy),
        121–22, 226–27
    Drumstick (Original
        Recipe), 121, 226–27
    Fajita Pita, 119, 198, 225
    Fil-A Sandwich, 194
    Fillet Biscuit, 114
    Giardino, 134–36, 238–39
    Grilled Breast Dinner,
        210–11

Grilled Ficelle Sandwich
  with Swiss, 177
Grilled Sandwich, 85, 168,
  200, 274
Grilled Sandwich with
  Cheese, 167, 275
Grilled Sourdough Club
  Sandwich, 224
Guiltless Grill Pita, 82
Guiltless Grill Sandwich,
  82
Half Frontega Panini,
  245–46
Half Italian Panini, 215,
  218
Half-size, 57–60
Honey BBQ Sandwich, 121
Italian Panini, 109
Krispy Tender Strips, 84
Leg, 111, 113
Leg, Fried, 221
Leg Meal, 85, 198–99
Leg with Gravy, 116
Low-Carb Charbroiled
  Grilled Club, 117
Margarita Grilled, 195–98
McGrill Sandwich, 133, 235
McNuggets, 130, 236
with Mushrooms, 142, 242
One-Fourth Dark Meal,
  182–84, 186–87
One-Fourth White Meal,
  184–85
Original Sandwich, 75
Pieces (2), 228–31
Popcorn, 219
Popcorn (Kid's Size), 122
with Potato, 244
Roast Breast with Sundried
  Tomato on Croissant,
  177
Roast Club Sandwich, 174
Sandwich Meal, 195

Sizzling Skillet, 59–60, 173
Small Club Sandwich, 259
Small Fiesta Sandwich, 260
Spicy Sandwich, 273
Spicy with Peanuts, 142,
  242, 244
Stars, 77, 192–93
with String Beans, 142,
  242, 244
Strip Dinner, 106
Strip Dinner (seniors only),
  211–12
Strips, 65, 80, 96
Strips, Crispy, 65, 171, 227
Super Bird Sandwich,
  99–100
Swiss, on Croissant, 63
Taquitos with Beans, 65
Tender Crisp Sandwich,
  121
Tender Roast Sandwich,
  121–22
Tenders, 75, 189–90
Tender Strips, Krispy, 199
Thigh, 113
Thigh Meal, 85, 200
Twister Wrap, 122
Two Pieces, 123
White, 68–71
Whopper, 74, 190
Whopper with Mayo, 74
Wing Meal, 84, 198–99
Wings, 199
Wings, Extra Crispy, 122
Wings, Honey BBQ, 121
Wrap with Brie, 63
Chick-fil-A, 79–80, 194–95
Chili
  Bowl, 197
  Carne Asada with Pinto
    Beans, 151
  Chicken with Black Beans,
    151

Chicken with Pinto Beans, 151
Large with Cheese, 275
Small, no Cheese, 168–69
Small with Cheese, 167, 274
Small with Double Cheese, 274
Turkey Cup, 217
Chili's, 80–83, 195–98
Cholesterol, 16–18
Chronic diseases, 16
Church's Chicken, 84–85, 198–200
Club Sandwich, 101
Cookies, 152, 157, 257, 262–63
Corn, 45
Corned beef. See Reuben
Cup, estimating, 42

Dairy Queen, 85, 200–201
Del Taco, 86–87, 201–202
Denny's, 87–106, 203–12
Dressing, 43
Drinks, 38–39

Eggbeaters, 88–96
with Cheese (2), 203–205
Eggs
Au Bon Pain, 62
Bacon & Cheese Biscuit, 125–26
and Bacon Frittata, 107
and Bacon on Spinach & Cheese Croissant, 177
on Bagel with Cheese, 176
on Bagel with Cheese and Bacon, 176–77
with Cheddar and Bacon on Croissant, 176
with Cheese (1), 203–206
Denny's Breakfast, 88–96
Denver Omelette, 107

Fat-Free on Spinach Bagel with Swiss, 176
Frittata, 212
Frittata Santa Fe, 107
Frittata with American Cheese, 213–14
Frittata with Cheddar Cheese, 214
Frittata with Provolone Cheese, 213–14
Frittata with Sausage, 214
Frittata with Swiss Cheese, 213
McMuffin, 126–29, 232–34
"Naked" Ham Frittata, 213
Patties (2), 188
Patty, 72
with Provolone Cheese, 176
Scrambled, 125, 127–28, 191, 232–33
Scrambled, Side, 76–77, 191–92
on Spinach and Cheese Croissant, 176
Tortilla Scrambler, 114, 220
Two, 203
Einstein Bros. Bagels, 106–10, 212–18
El Pollo Loco, 111–13, 218–20
Emotional overeating, 50–52
Enchilada
Chicken, 65–66
Verano, 179
Enchirito
Chicken, 161, 269
Steak, 161
Extra food, 45–46

Fad diets, 1
Fat, 10–11, 16–18
Fish. See also Seafood; Shrimp; Tuna

Baja Taco, 65, 67
and Chips, 106
Half Catfish, 149
Half Red Snapper, 147–48
Half Salmon, 148
Half Tilapia, 147
Half Trout, 148
Jack Daniel's Salmon, 162, 270
One Piece, 123
Salmon, Ginger-Citrus Glazed, 83
Salmon Dinner, Atlantic Baked, 140–41
Three-Fourths Catfish Meal, 252
Tilapia with Mango Salsa, 56, 172
Two-Thirds Trout Meal, 252
Two-Thirds Salmon Meal, 251
Two-Thirds Snapper Meal, 251
Two-Thirds Tilapia Meal, 250
40–30–30 meal, 3–7, 20–21
French, 18–19
French Dip Sub, 61

Golden Gate Gourmet Sandwich, 68, 180
Grains, 7, 9

Ham
Big Hot 'N Cheese Sandwich, 116, 222
Black Forest on Challah, 109–10
and Cheese Croissant, 114–15
and Cheese Meal, 271
and Cheese Panini, 108
and Cheese Sandwich, 165
and Cheese Small Original Sandwich, 259
Croissant with Cheese, 72
Croissant with Egg, 72
and Double Egg Sandwich with Cheese, 261
Egg, and Cheese Biscuit, 113
Egg, Cheese Croissant, 73, 187–88
Egg, Cheese Sourdough Sandwich, 73, 188
and Egg Sandwich with Cheese, 155–56
Half Black Forest on Challah, 216–17
Half & Cheese Panini, 217
Half Smoked & Swiss on Rye, 143, 145
Hot & Cheese Sandwich, 60, 221
Meal, 183
on Rye, 207–208
Sourdough Sandwich, 76, 191
Sub with Cheese, 68
with Sundried Tomato on Croissant, 178
Sunrise Croissant, 114–15, 220
Swiss, Sandwich, 60
and Swiss on Rye, 98, 100
and Swiss on Rye (seniors only), 207
and Turkey Meal, 271
and Turkey Sandwich, 165
Hamburger. *See also* Cheeseburger; Veggie burger
A&W, 65, 171
A&W Deluxe, 65

Bacon Cheddar (seniors only), 207
Big 'N Tasty, 132
Big 'N Tasty with Cheese, 235
BK, 190
Chili, 77
Classic, 98, 209
Classic Single, 167–68, 273
Classic Single with Cheese, 273, 275
Deluxe, 169, 171
Deluxe with Chili, 169
Double, 75, 189
Double-Double, 223
Double Meat, 117, 222–224
with Extra Meat, 118
Famous Star, 77–78
Famous Star with Cheese, 193–94
Grilled Sourdough with Bacon and Onions, 115
Grilled Sourdough with Swiss Cheese and Onions, 116
In-N-Out, 223
Kid's, 168
Oldtimer, 82
Original, 169
Original with Chili, 170
Protein-Style Double Meat, 117–18, 222–23
Quarter Pounder with Cheese, 234, 237
Sourdough Bacon, 192
Whopper, 189–90
Whopper Jr., 190
Whopper Jr. with Cheese, 73, 189
Whopper with Cheese, Bacon, 73
Wienerschnitzel Meal, 277
Hardee's, 113–17, 220–22

Heart disease, 16–18
Hunger between meals, 47–49
Hunter-gatherer diet, 7, 9–10

In-N-Out, 117–18, 222–23
Insulin, 12–13, 16
Italians, 15

Jack in the Box, 118–20, 224–26

KFC (Kentucky Fried Chicken), 120–22, 226–27

Leptin, 10
Lettuce Wraps, 81, 198
Long John Silver's, 123–25, 228–31
Low-carb diet, 8
Lox and Cream Cheese Sandwich, 107

McDonald's, 125–34, 231–38
Meatloaf
  Boston Market, 182–183
  Half-size, 70
Melt
  Albacore Tuna, 97, 259
  Dijon Horseradish, 160
  Dijon Horseradish with Double Cheese, 265
  Steak & Onion, 67, 180
  Subway, 160
Men's meals
  Applebee's, 172–74
  Arby's, 174–75
  Au Bon Pain, 176–78
  A&W, 171–72
  Baja Fresh, 178–80
  Blimpie, 180–82
  Boston Market, 182–87
  Burger King, 187–90

Carl's Jr., 191–94
Chick-fil-A, 194–95
Chili's, 195–98
Church's Chicken, 198–200
Dairy Queen, 200–201
Del Taco, 201–202
Denny's, 203–12
Einstein Bros. Bagels, 212–18
El Pollo Loco, 218–20
Hardee's, 220–22
In-N-Out, 222–23
Jack in the Box, 224–26
KFC, 226–27
Long John Silver's, 228–31
McDonald's, 231–38
Olive Garden, 238–39
Outback Steakhouse, 240–42
Panda Express, 242–44
Panera Bread, 244–47
Pizza Hut, 247–50
Red Lobster, 250–52
Rubio's Fresh Mexican Grill, 253–56
Schlotzky's Deli, 257–60
Subway, 261–67
Taco Bell, 268–69
TGI Friday's, 269–70
Togo's, 271–72
Wendy's, 272–75
Wienerschnitzel, 276–77
Menus, 25–29
Milk, 37–38

Net carbs, 26
Nuts, 33–35

Olive Garden, 134–36, 238–39
Onion Rings, 78
Outback Steakhouse, 136–41, 240–42
Overeating, 15–16, 49–52

Panda Express, 141–42, 242–44
Panera Bread, 143–45, 244–47
Pannido
  Deli Trio Sandwich, 224
  Ham & Turkey, 226
Pasta, 15
Pastrami
  Half Small Reuben, 154
  Half Small & Swiss, 154
  Sandwich, 181
  and Swiss Sandwich, 153
Personal Pan Pizza, 145–46, 248–50
Philly Cheesesteak Sandwich, 120, 226
Philly Sandwich, 155
Pizza Hut, 145–46, 247–50
Portion sizes, 30–31
Portobello & Mozzarella Panini, 145
Pot Roast
  Dinner (seniors only), 211
  with Gravy, 104–105
Protein, 12–15, 35–37

Quesadilla
  Chicken, 112, 220
  Chicken Cheddar, 202
  Chicken Fajita, 83
  Spicy Jack, 202
  Steak, 66

Red Lobster, 147–49, 250–52
Reuben
  Grilled, 181
  Small, 260
  Small Turkey, 260
Ribs
  Grilled Baby Back with Cinnamon Apples, 81

Roast Beef
  Big Sandwich, 221
  and Cheese Sandwich, 155
  Giant Sandwich, 175
  Half Asiago Sandwich, 246
  Half Sandwich with
    Cheddar, Swiss, and
    Sundried Tomato, 177
  Regular Sandwich, 115, 175
Roast beef
  Sandwich, 60
  Sandwich with Cheddar, 63
Rubio's Fresh Mexican Grill,
  149–51, 253–256

Salad, 40–45
  Asian Chicken, 119, 225
  Asian Sesame, 60–61, 175,
    245
  Caesar, 57–60, 134
  Chicken, Charbroiled,
    78–79
  Chicken, Crispy, 85, 229,
    231
  Chicken, Grilled, 85,
    200–201
  Chicken, Oriental Grilled,
    70
  Chicken Breast, Grilled, 97,
    100, 208–209
  Chicken Caesar, 74–75,
    153–54, 163–64, 173–74,
    219, 241–42, 246, 258,
    269–70
  Chicken Caesar, Crispy, 129
  Chicken Caesar, Grilled,
    83, 133–34
  Chicken Caesar, Half-Size,
    173–74
  Chicken Caesar, Small
    Chicken Portion, 136–38
  Chicken Caribbean,
    Grilled, 83

Chicken Chipotle, 110, 217
Chicken Club, 118, 175
Chicken Garden,
  Chargrilled, 79
Chicken Sandwich, 195,
  246
Chicken Strip, 101–102
Chicken Strip, Fried, 209
Chinese Chicken, 153
Classic Cafe, 245–246
Cobb, California, 129–30
Crispy Chicken Bacon
  Ranch, 236, 238
Dinner Caesar, 80–81
Fiesta, 131–32, 236
Grilled Chopped Chicken,
  151
Half Asian Sesame
  Chicken, 144
Half Classic Cafe, 144
Half Cobbie on Challah,
  216
Half Grilled Chicken
  Caesar, 145
HealthMex Chicken,
  255–56
Mandarin Chicken, 167,
  273
Martha's Vineyard,
  174–175
Mediterranean Chicken,
  158, 263
Mediterranean with Roast
  Beef, 159
Shrimp Caesar, 75, 138–39,
  141, 240
Shrimp & Seafood, 124–25,
  228–31
Side, 131–32, 236–37
Smoked Turkey Chef's,
  154, 259–60
Southwest Chicken, 119,
  195, 225

Spring Mix, 167
Taco, 162, 268
Taco Supremo with Salsa,
274–275
Tostada, 219
Tuna Sandwich (seniors
only), 207
Turkey Breast, 97
Salami
Capicolla, Mortadella,
Cotta Sandwich, 166,
271
Italian Dry and Cheese,
272
Salsa, 111, 150, 218, 253
Saturated fats, 16–17
Sausage
McMuffin with Egg,
231–32
Sourdough Sandwich,
192
Schlotzky's Deli, 152–55,
257–60
Seafood. See Fish; Shrimp;
Tuna
Sears, Barry, Ph.D, 2, 20,
279
7-Day Quick-Start Diet,
29–31
drinks, 38–39
emotional overeating,
50–52
extra food, 45–46
how to follow, 31–32
hunger between meals,
47–49
salads, 40–45
snacks, 32–38
tips for weight loss, 52–53
vitamins, 39–40
Shrimp
Fried (7), 103–104
Fried Dinner, 104, 212

Primavera, 135, 239
Taco, 65
Teriyaki Skewers, 56–57,
172
Slammer, 221
with Cheese, 116, 221–22
Smart-Carb Guide
drinks, 38–39
emotional overeating,
50–52
extra food, 45–46
getting started, 21–22
hunger between meals,
47–49
men's meals, 171–277
menus, 25–28
restaurant low-carb menus,
28–29
salads, 40–45
7-Day Quick-Start Diet,
29–32
snacks, 32–38
tips for weight loss, 52–53
using, 23–25
vitamins, 39–40
women's meals, 55–170
Snacks, 32–38
Soup
Bowl Tortilla, 83
Chicken Enchilada, 80–81,
197
Chicken Tortilla, 82–83
Low-Fat Chicken Noodle,
145
Low-Fat Vegetable Garden,
144
Vegetable Beef, 99
Vegetarian Black Bean,
144
South Beach Diet, 20
Splitting meals, 27–28
Steak
Chilito Taco, 64

and Egg Sandwich with
  Cheese, 155–56
and Egg Sandwich with
  Double Cheese, 261
Onion Melt, 67
Sirloin, 105–106, 163
Sirloin Dinner, 210
Sirloin Dinner with Potato,
  139–40, 240–41, 269
String Beans with Fried Tofu,
  244
Sub
  BBQ Pulled Pork, 265
  Blimpie's Best, 181
  Buffalo Chicken, 160
  Cheese Steak, 159, 264
  Chicken Breast, 160
  Chicken Breast with
    Cheese, 266
  Club with Cheese, 68
  Cold Cut Combo with
    Double Cheese, 264
  French Dip, 61, 174
  Grilled Chicken with
    Mayo, 181
  Ham with Cheese, 68, 181,
    267
  Ham with Cheese and
    Bacon, 159
  Ham with Double Cheese,
    161, 266
  Ham with Double Meat,
    266
  Ham with Extra Cheese,
    182
  Meatball, 272
  Mediterranean Chicken,
    265
  Poblano Cheddar Turkey
    with Double Cheese,
    265
  Roast Beef with Cheese,
    159, 267
Roast Beef with Double
  Cheese, 265
Roast Beef with Double
  Meat, 264
Savory Chicken Caesar,
  265
Seafood and Crab with
  Double Cheese, 158
Steak and Double Cheese,
  264
Subway Club, 160
Subway Club with Cheese,
  266
Subway Melt with Double
  Cheese, 264
Sweet Onion Chicken with
  Cheese, 264
Tuna with Cheese, 68
Turkey and Ham with
  Cheese, 159
Turkey and Ham with
  Double Cheese, 266
Turkey with Cheese, 68,
  267
Turkey with Cheese and
  Bacon, 159
Turkey with Double
  Cheese, 160, 266
Turkey with Double Meat,
  266
Turkey with Extra Cheese,
  182
Turkey with Extra Swiss,
  181
Turkey with Swiss and
  Provolone, 181
Subway, 155–61, 261–67
Sugar coma, 12
Super Bird Sandwich,
  208

Tablespoon, estimating,
  43

Taco
  Baja Fish, 65, 67
  Carne Asada, 151, 253–55
  Carnitas, 87, 202
  Chicken, 179
  Chicken al Carbon, 219
  Chicken Chilito, 64
  Chicken Del Carbon,
    86–87, 201
  Chicken Soft, 86–87,
    161–62, 219, 268–69
  Fish, 64, 66
  Fresco Style, 161, 268–69
  Grilled Chicken, 255–56
  Grilled Fish, 151, 255–256
  HealthMex with Chicken,
    151, 254–55
  Shrimp, 65
  Steak, 64, 178–80
  Steak Chilito, 64
  Steak Del Carbon, 87,
    201–202
  Street Carne Asada, 150–51
  Street Carnitas, 150–51,
    253–55
  Ultimate, 87
Taco Bell, 161–62, 268–69
Taquitos
  Chicken with Beans, 65
TGI Friday's, 162–64,
    269–70
Togo's, 164–66, 271–72
Tortilla Scrambler, 114, 220
Tostadita
  Steak Mini, 180
Trans-fatty acids, 17
Tuna
  Albacore on Artisan Bread,
    108, 110, 215–17
  Albacore Sandwich, 166,
    271
  Cheddar, on Croissant, 63
  Margarita Grilled, 196

Turkey
  on Asiago Cheese Bagel,
    109
  and Bacon Small Club, 260
  Bowl Chili, 108
  Breast, Half-Size, 69–70
  Breast, Ham & Bacon
    Melt, 265
  Breast on Whole Wheat,
    101, 209
  and Brie, on Bagel, 63
  and Cheese Meal, 271
  and Cheese Sandwich, 165
  Half Breast Meal, 185–86
  Half Carver Sandwich, 70
  Half Roasted on Artisan
    Bread, 215–16
  Half Sandwich, 82, 197
  Half Sandwich on
    Multigrain, 218
  Half Smoked Breast on
    Sourdough, 245
  Half Smoked Breast
    Sandwich, 143–44
  Half Smokehouse Panini
    on Focaccia, 247
  Half Tasty on Asiago
    Cheese Bagel, 215
  and Ham with Cheese, 272
  Roasted Sandwich, 120, 225
  Sandwich on Artisan
    Wheat Bread, 108, 110
  Small Guacamole
    Sandwich, 155
  Small Original Sandwich,
    260
  with Stuffing and Gravy,
    102–103
  Zesty Pannido Sandwich,
    118

Ultimate Club Sandwich, 120,
  225

Veggie burger
  BK, 73, 189
  BK with Cheese, 73
Vitamins, 39–40

Weight loss, 19–21
  menus for, 25–29
  methods for, 23–25
  tips for, 52–53
Wendy's, 166–169, 272–275
Wienerschnitzel, 169–70,
    276–77
Women's meals
  Applebee's, 56–60
  Arby's, 60–61
  Au Bon Pain, 61–63
  A&W, 55–56
  Baja Fresh, 64–67
  Blimpie, 67–68
  Boston Market, 68–71
  Burger King, 72–75
  Carl's Jr., 76–79
  Chick-fil-A, 79–80
  Chili's, 80–83
  Church's Chicken, 84–85
  Dairy Queen, 85
  Del Taco, 86–87
  Denny's, 87–106
  Einstein Bros. Bagels,
    106–10
  El Pollo Loco, 111–13
  Hardee's, 113–17
  In-N-Out, 117–18
  Jack in the Box, 118–20
  KFC, 120–22

  Long John Silver's, 123–25
  McDonald's, 125–34
  Olive Garden, 134–36
  Outback Steakhouse,
    136–41
  Panda Express, 141–42
  Panera Bread, 143–45
  Pizza Hut, 145–46
  Red Lobster, 147–49
  Rubio's Fresh Mexican
    Grill, 149–51
  Schlotzky's Deli, 152–55
  Subway, 155–61
  Taco Bell, 161–62
  TGI Friday's, 162–64
  Togo's, 164–66
  Wendy's, 166–69
  Wienerschnitzel, 169–70
Wrap
  Chicken Caesar with Brie,
    63
  Salsa Chicken with
    Cheddar, 259
  Seafood & Crab, 159,
    263–64
  Turkey and Cheese, 265–66
  Turkey with Swiss, 63
  Veggie Delight with
    Double Cheese, 158
  Veggie Delight with Triple
    Cheese, 267

Yogurt, 37–38

Zone Diet, 2–3, 20, 279

The 7-Day Quick-Start Diet for WOMEN

DAY 1: Arby's Day

MEAL	EAT

BREAKFAST

Arby's may not be open for breakfast. Instead, go to McDonald's and order:

> Scrambled Eggs
> 2 pieces Canadian Bacon
> Hash Browns
> Apple Dippers (no dipping sauce)
> Optional: 1 packet ketchup on the eggs

LUNCH Regular Roast Beef Sandwich

SNACK SMART-CARB SNACK

DINNER Hot Ham 'n Cheese Sandwich

SNACK SMART-CARB SNACK

DAY 2: Burger King Day

MEAL	EAT
BREAKFAST	Croissant with Ham and Egg Sandwich (extra ham, no cheese)
LUNCH	Whopper Jr. with Cheese (no mayo)
SNACK	SMART-CARB SNACK
DINNER	Chicken Garden Salad (no Parmesan cheese) Garlic Cheese Toast (comes with salad) ¾ packet Tomato Balsamic Vinaigrette Dressing
SNACK	SMART-CARB SNACK

DAY 3: KFC Day

MEAL	EAT
BREAKFAST	

KFC may not be open for breakfast. Instead, go to McDonald's and order:

Scrambled Eggs

Chocolate Milk
Optional: 1 packet ketchup on the
eggs

LUNCH	Honey BBQ Chicken Sandwich (discard ¼ the bread—take it from the bottom)
SNACK	SMART-CARB SNACK
DINNER	Drumstick (Original Recipe) Macaroni & Cheese Small Corn* Note: Hold the biscuit
SNACK	SMART-CARB SNACK

*If the restaurant doesn't offer the small corn (3 inches), eat
½ the large corn (5½ inches).

DAY 4: McDonald's Day

MEAL	**EAT**
BREAKFAST	Egg McMuffin with extra egg
LUNCH	Big 'N Tasty (no mayo, discard the bottom piece of bread)

SNACK   SMART-CARB SNACK

DINNER   Grilled Chicken Caesar Salad
              (remove ½ the chicken)
              ½ packet Low-Fat Balsamic
              Vinaigrette Dressing
              Snack-Sized Fruit & Yogurt Parfait
              (discard the granola)*

SNACK   SMART-CARB SNACK

*You can order the Reduced-Fat Vanilla Ice Cream Cone (eat the cone) instead of the Fruit & Yogurt Parfait. Leftover chicken from the salad can be used for making snacks (see page 32). Extra chicken = 2 Proteins

DAY 5: Subway Day

How to Order Your Sub:

+ Bread: any
+ Vegetables: any
+ Cheese: Swiss, provolone, or Cheddar
+ Condiments (optional): salt, pepper, vinegar, mustard

Tip:

+ Don't add mayo or olive oil to the sub.

MEAL	EAT
BREAKFAST	Cheese & Egg Breakfast Sandwich with double cheese (discard ¼ the bread)*
LUNCH	6-inch Cheese Steak Sub (discard ¼ the bread)
SNACK	SMART-CARB SNACK
DINNER	Mediterranean Chicken Salad (no dressing) Red Wine Vinaigrette Dressing (on the side—use the whole container) 1 package croutons (comes with salad)
SNACK	SMART-CARB SNACK

*If the Subway near you doesn't serve breakfast, order the foot-long Cheese Steak Sub. Eat half for breakfast and half for lunch (discard ¼ the bread before eating).

DAY 6: Taco Bell Day

Have as much taco sauce as you like.

MEAL	EAT
BREAKFAST	

Taco Bell may not be open for breakfast. Instead, go to McDonald's and order:

Scrambled Eggs
Cheese (on the eggs)
Snack-Sized Fruit & Yogurt Parfait
(discard the granola)

LUNCH   Crunchy Taco
Chicken Soft Taco (Fresco Style)

SNACK   SMART-CARB SNACK

DINNER   Chicken Enchirito

SNACK   SMART-CARB SNACK

DAY 7: Wendy's Day

MEAL   **EAT**
BREAKFAST
Wendy's may not be open for breakfast. Instead, go to
McDonald's and order:

Bacon, Egg & Cheese Biscuit (no
bacon, discard ¼ of the bread)
2 pieces Canadian Bacon
Optional: 1 packet ketchup

LUNCH   Classic Single (no mayo, no cheese,
discard ¼ the bread)

SNACK   SMART-CARB SNACK

DINNER   Small Chili (no cheese, no crackers)
                 Side Salad (no croutons)
                 ½ packet Caesar Dressing

SNACK   SMART-CARB SNACK

The 7-Day
Quick-Start
Diet for
MEN

DAY 1: Arby's Day

MEAL	EAT

BREAKFAST

Arby's may not be open for breakfast. Instead, go to McDonald's and order:

Egg McMuffin (extra Canadian bacon, extra cheese)

LUNCH — Giant Roast Beef Sandwich

SNACK — SMART-CARB SNACK

DINNER — Roast Chicken Club Sandwich (no mayo)

SNACK — SMART-CARB SNACK

DAY 2: Burger King Day

Meal	Eat
Breakfast	Croissant with Ham, Egg, & Cheese Sandwich (extra ham, extra cheese) 1 packet ketchup (on sandwich)
Lunch	Whopper (no mayo, discard ¼ the bread)
Snack	SMART-CARB SNACK
Dinner	Chicken Garden Salad (no Garlic Parmesan Toast) Fat-Free Ranch Dressing ¾ Small Fries* 1 packet ketchup (optional)
Snack	SMART-CARB SNACK

*If they don't offer Small Fries, order Medium Fries and eat half. To avoid eating the rest, discard them before beginning your meal.

DAY 3: KFC Day

Meal	Eat

Breakfast

KFC may not be open for breakfast. Instead, go to McDonald's and order:

> Bacon, Egg & Cheese Biscuit with extra cheese
> Canadian Bacon (side order)

Lunch

> Drumstick (Original Recipe)
> Drumstick (Extra Crispy)
> Biscuit (no butter)

Snack

SMART-CARB SNACK

Dinner

> Drumstick (Extra Crispy)
> Wing (Original Recipe)
> Large Corn*
> Note: Hold the Biscuit

Snack

SMART-CARB SNACK

*If the restaurant doesn't offer the large corn (5½ inches), order two small corns (3 inches).

DAY 4: McDonald's Day

MEAL	EAT
BREAKFAST	Sausage McMuffin with Egg
LUNCH	Big 'N Tasty with Cheese (no mayo)
SNACK	SMART-CARB SNACK
DINNER	Crispy Chicken Bacon Ranch Salad (no croutons, no dressing) ½ packet Low-Fat Balsamic Vinaigrette Dressing
SNACK	SMART-CARB SNACK

DAY 5: Subway Day

How to Order Your Sandwich:

+ Bread: any
+ Vegetables: any
+ Cheese: Swiss, provolone, or Cheddar
+ Condiments (optional): salt, pepper, vinegar, mustard

Tip:

+ Don't add mayo or olive oil to the sub.

MEAL	EAT
BREAKFAST	Bacon & Egg Breakfast Sandwich (add cheese, extra egg)*
LUNCH	6-inch Cheese Steak Sub with extra cheese
SNACK	SMART-CARB SNACK
DINNER	Mediterranean Chicken Salad with Croutons (no dressing) Oil and vinegar (on the salad) Lay's Original *Baked* Potato Chips
SNACK	SMART-CARB SNACK

*If the Subway near you doesn't serve breakfast sandwiches, order the footlong Cheese Steak Sub with extra cheese. Eat half for breakfast and half for lunch.

DAY 6: Taco Bell Day

You can have as much taco sauce as you like.

MEAL   **EAT**

BREAKFAST

Taco Bell may not be open for breakfast. Instead, go to
McDonald's and order:

> Scrambled Eggs (side order)
> 2 orders Bacon (4 pieces)
> English Muffin (no butter)
> 1 packet ketchup
> Tip: Make everything into a
> sandwich.

LUNCH   Chicken Soft Taco
                Steak Soft Taco

SNACK   SMART-CARB SNACK

DINNER   Taco Salad (no sour cream, discard $2/3$
                of the shell)

SNACK   SMART-CARB SNACK

DAY 7: Wendy's Day

MEAL	EAT

BREAKFAST

Wendy's may not be open for breakfast. Instead, go to McDonald's and order:

> Scrambled Eggs
> Canadian Bacon
> Hash Browns
> Chocolate Milk
> Optional: 1 packet ketchup

LUNCH Classic Single with Cheese (no mayo)

SNACK SMART-CARB SNACK

DINNER Taco Supremo Salad with Salsa (no sour cream, no chips)

SNACK SMART-CARB SNACK

The 7-Day Quick-Start Diet for WOMEN

DAY 1: Arby's Day

BREAKFAST Arby's may not be open for breakfast. Instead, go to McDonald's and order: Scrambled Eggs, 2 pieces Canadian Bacon, Hash Browns, Apple Dippers (no dipping sauce). Optional: 1 packet ketchup on the eggs

LUNCH Regular Roast Beef Sandwich

SNACK SMART-CARB SNACK

DINNER Hot Ham 'n Cheese Sandwich

SNACK SMART-CARB SNACK

DAY 2: Burger King Day

BREAKFAST Croissant with Ham and Egg Sandwich (extra ham, no cheese)

LUNCH Whopper Jr. with Cheese (no mayo)

SNACK SMART-CARB SNACK

DINNER Chicken Garden Salad (no Parmesan cheese), Garlic Cheese Toast (comes with salad), $3/4$ packet Tomato Balsamic Vinaigrette Dressing

SNACK SMART-CARB SNACK

DAY 3: KFC Day

BREAKFAST KFC may not be open for breakfast. Instead, go to McDonald's and order: Scrambled Eggs, Chocolate Milk. Optional: 1 packet ketchup on the eggs

LUNCH Honey BBQ Chicken Sandwich (discard $1/4$ the bread—take it from the bottom)

SNACK SMART-CARB SNACK

DINNER Drumstick (Original Recipe), Macaroni & Cheese, Small Corn*
Note: Hold the biscuit

SNACK SMART-CARB SNACK

*If the restaurant doesn't offer the small corn (3 inches), eat $1/2$ the large corn ($5\frac{1}{2}$ inches).

DAY 4: McDonald's Day

BREAKFAST Egg McMuffin with extra egg

LUNCH Big 'N Tasty (no mayo, discard the bottom piece of bread)

SNACK SMART-CARB SNACK

DINNER Grilled Chicken Caesar Salad (remove $1/2$ the chicken), $1/2$ packet Low-Fat Balsamic Vinaigrette Dressing, Snack-Sized Fruit & Yogurt Parfait (discard the granola)*

SNACK SMART-CARB SNACK

*You can order the Reduced-Fat Vanilla Ice Cream Cone (eat the cone) instead of the Fruit & Yogurt Parfait. Leftover chicken from the salad can be used for making snacks (see pg. 32). Extra chicken = 2 Proteins

DAY 5: Subway Day

How to Order Your Sub:

+ Bread: any
+ Vegetables: any
+ Cheese: Swiss, provolone, or Cheddar
+ Condiments (optional): salt, pepper, vinegar, mustard

Tip:

+ Don't add mayo or olive oil to the sub.

BREAKFAST Cheese & Egg Breakfast Sandwich with double cheese (discard $\frac{1}{4}$ the bread)*

LUNCH 6-inch Cheese Steak Sub (discard $\frac{1}{4}$ the bread)

SNACK SMART-CARB SNACK

DINNER Mediterranean Chicken Salad (no dressing), Red Wine Vinaigrette Dressing (on the side—use the whole container), 1 package croutons (comes with salad)

SNACK SMART-CARB SNACK

*If the Subway near you doesn't serve breakfast, order the foot-long Cheese Steak Sub. Eat half for breakfast and half for lunch (discard $\frac{1}{4}$ the bread before eating).

DAY 6: Taco Bell Day

Have as much taco sauce as you like.

BREAKFAST Taco Bell may not be open for breakfast. Instead, go to McDonald's and order: Scrambled Eggs, Cheese (on the eggs), Snack-Sized Fruit & Yogurt Parfait (discard the granola)

LUNCH Crunchy Taco Chicken Soft Taco (Fresco Style)

SNACK SMART-CARB SNACK

DINNER Chicken Enchirito

SNACK SMART-CARB SNACK

DAY 7: Wendy's Day

BREAKFAST Wendy's may not be open for breakfast. Instead, go to McDonald's and order: Bacon, Egg & Cheese Biscuit (no bacon, discard $\frac{1}{4}$ of the bread), 2 pieces Canadian Bacon. Optional: 1 packet ketchup

LUNCH Classic Single (no mayo, no cheese, discard $\frac{1}{4}$ the bread)

SNACK SMART-CARB SNACK

DINNER Small Chili (no cheese, no crackers), Side Salad (no croutons), $\frac{1}{2}$ packet Caesar Dressing

SNACK SMART-CARB SNACK

The 7-Day Quick-Start Diet for MEN

DAY 1: Arby's Day

BREAKFAST Arby's may not be open for breakfast. Instead, go to McDonald's and order: Egg McMuffin (extra Canadian bacon, extra cheese)

LUNCH Giant Roast Beef Sandwich

SNACK SMART-CARB SNACK

DINNER Roast Chicken Club Sandwich (no mayo)

SNACK SMART-CARB SNACK

DAY 2: Burger King Day

BREAKFAST Croissant with Ham, Egg, & Cheese Sandwich (extra ham, extra cheese), 1 packet ketchup (on sandwich)

LUNCH Whopper (no mayo, discard ¼ the bread)

SNACK SMART-CARB SNACK

DINNER Chicken Garden Salad (no Garlic Parmesan Toast), Fat Free Ranch Dressing, ¾ Small Fries*, 1 packet ketchup (optional)

SNACK SMART-CARB SNACK

*If they don't offer Small Fries, order Medium Fries and eat half. To avoid eating the rest, discard them before beginning your meal.

DAY 3: KFC Day

BREAKFAST KFC may not be open for breakfast. Instead, go to McDonald's and order: Bacon, Egg & Cheese Biscuit with extra cheese, Canadian Bacon (side order)

LUNCH Drumstick (Original Recipe), Drumstick (Extra Crispy), Biscuit (no butter)

SNACK SMART-CARB SNACK

DINNER Drumstick (Extra Crispy), Wing (Original Recipe), Large Corn*
Note: Hold the biscuit

SNACK SMART-CARB SNACK

*If the restaurant doesn't offer the large corn (5½ inches), order two small corns (3 inches).

DAY 4: McDonald's Day

BREAKFAST Sausage McMuffin with Egg

LUNCH Big 'N Tasty with Cheese (no mayo)

SNACK SMART-CARB SNACK

DINNER Crispy Chicken Bacon Ranch Salad (no croutons, no dressing), ½ packet Low-Fat Balsamic Vinaigrette Dressing

SNACK SMART-CARB SNACK

DAY 5: Subway Day

How to Order Your Sandwich:

+ Bread: any
+ Vegetables: any
+ Cheese: Swiss, provolone, or cheddar
+ Condiments (optional): salt, pepper, vinegar, mustard

Tip:

+ Don't add mayo or olive oil to the sub.

BREAKFAST Bacon & Egg Breakfast Sandwich (add cheese, extra egg)*
LUNCH 6-inch Cheese Steak Sub with extra cheese
SNACK SMART-CARB SNACK
DINNER Mediterranean Chicken Salad with Croutons (no dressing), oil and vinegar (on the salad), Lay's Original *Baked* Potato Chips
SNACK SMART-CARB SNACK

*If the Subway near you doesn't serve breakfast sandwiches, order the foot-long Cheese Steak Sub with extra cheese. Eat half for breakfast and half for lunch.

DAY 6: Taco Bell Day

You can have as much taco sauce as you like.

BREAKFAST Taco Bell may not be open for breakfast. Instead, go to McDonald's and order: Scrambled Eggs (side order), 2 orders Bacon (4 pieces), English Muffin (no butter), 1 packet ketchup. Tip: Make everything into a sandwich.
LUNCH Chicken Soft Taco, Steak Soft Taco
SNACK SMART-CARB SNACK
DINNER Taco Salad (no sour cream, discard $2/3$ of the shell)
SNACK SMART-CARB SNACK

DAY 7: Wendy's Day

BREAKFAST Wendy's may not be open for breakfast. Instead, go to McDonald's and order: Scrambled Eggs, Canadian Bacon, Hash Browns, Chocolate Milk. Optional: 1 packet ketchup
LUNCH Classic Single with Cheese (no mayo)
SNACK SMART-CARB SNACK
DINNER Taco Supremo Salad with Salsa (no sour cream, no chips)
SNACK SMART-CARB SNACK